FEMALE MUTILATION

A global journey behind the curtains of the horrifying worldwide practice of female genital mutilation

D1340032

Hilary Burrage

NEW
HOLLAND

Contents

(The Questionnaire used throughout can be found on the *Female Mutilation Worldwide* website under Further Reading)

"This book is most welcome. Each page …. rings the bell of the rebellion against female genital mutilation."
Dr. Morissanda Kouyaté Executive Director of the Inter-African Committee

PREFACE

'Yet another book on female genital mutilation?'

No. Millions of voices and millions of pages on Female Genital Mutilation (FGM) will never be enough to describe this practice, coming from the depths of time in order, as it is believed, to submit and control women's sexuality for the benefit of men.

To achieve this sole purpose many forms of unfounded justifications are put forward: women's cleanliness, purity of the female body, religious prescriptions, ritual passage to a superior social level, self-control, family honour, etc. The colour of the cast does not change the fracture. Regardless of the names and the forms given to FGM, the practice will always remain what it is: **mutilation**.

During the last thirty years, the biggest challenge for those who fight for the elimination of female genital mutilation has been to make the world understand, as this book demonstrates, that FGM is not an esoteric phenomenon belonging to African tribes lost in the African savannahs and forests, to whom the rest of humanity must pay absolute respect. On the contrary, it is a clear violation of the rights and the physical and psychological integrity of girls and women wherever the practice exists.

We are combating a harmful practice and not a culture, because culture is highly positive. It is important to dispel any ambiguity: female genital mutilation can in no way be considered an element of any culture, when it consists of cutting and scraping the female genital organs in the name of absurdity.

For the purpose of clarification and exhaustiveness, FGM has been classified in different types depending on the severity and depth of the mutilation. This classification, although academically interesting, cannot hide the fact that there is actually one single type, the one that damages girls and women in their flesh, no matter the depth of the cut, which sometimes ends in the almost total closure of the vagina.

So this book is most welcome. The idea that FGM is only an African practice is no longer valid, since wherever an ounce of human rights is violated the entire humanity must react.

The Protocol to the African Charter on Human and Peoples' Rights, on the Rights of Women, adopted by the African Heads of State in 2003 in Maputo, and *Resolution 67/146 of the United Nations General Assembly*, are examples of the global commitment against female genital mutilation. From Kenya to Australia, from Egypt to the United States of America, from the United Kingdom to Sierra Leone, from Uganda to Yemen, from France to Iraq, the mobilisation must be total in order to eradicate this backward and inhuman practice.

Aware of the immensity and universality of the fight against FGM, the Inter-African Committee on Traditional Practices Affecting the Health of Women and Children has set up, in addition to its 29 African national committees, 19 affiliated branches throughout the world, concentrating on 5 strategic axes: advocacy and sensitisation, legislation, retraining of excisers, care for victims and networking.

Each page in this book rings the bell of the rebellion against female genital mutilation.

Let us not comment on what it has taught us or try to find out who wrote it and for whom it is intended. The only question we should ask ourselves is:

What can I do to participate actively in this wonderful human adventure to free the world from one of the most absurd traditions, detrimental to the rights, the health and the life of women and girls?

Dr Morissanda Kouyaté

ACKNOWLEDGEMENTS

The many people who have contributed to this book are its very essence. I am deeply grateful to each and every one of you, for taking time to request and then return your completed questionnaires and for bearing with me whilst I despatched numerous emails asking endless questions. Thank you for trusting me to try to get it right.

Huge thanks is owed to everyone who provided material to construct a narrative or who agreed to be part of this endeavour in any other way. For some I know it has not been easy, but I hope very sincerely you will all feel that the effort has been worthwhile. Each contribution is unique, and each adds infinite value to the momentum towards our common goal, the eradication of female genital mutilation.

Thanks are also due to Diane Ward and the team at New Holland, for their determination that I should write this book, for agreeing that it should be such an ambitious project and, very importantly, for their faith and patience when eventually it took longer than we might have wished.

I must also thank my family, especially my mother, daughter and sister, and many of my friends for their support and fortitude as they lived this project with me. Neither the subject nor the exercise has been easy and I hope you already know that I am very grateful to you all.

Finally I want to thank my husband, Tony (Martin Anthony) Burrage, for his steadfast and generous encouragement, every day for many, many months, as he shared his time, attentive concern and resources to keep me going. Without him this assignment would quite simply never have been delivered.

Hilary Burrage
www.hilaryburrage.com
June 2015

Chapter 1:

FGM is Everyone's Business

This book comprises a collection of narratives by people whose lives have been touched, often very fundamentally, by female genital mutilation or, as many people call it, FGM.

The chapters of this book take us on a journey all around the world, across five continents. The stories are told by many and various people who offered, or whom I invited, to share their views and experiences, to help us all better understand what FGM 'means', and what campaigns and tactics are best suited, in what circumstances, to ensure that the practice is eradicated.

How can it possibly be that across the globe about 130, perhaps 140, million women and girls, even now alive, have endured and continue to live with the consequences of female genital mutilation?

And however can it be that, as things stand, some three million more girls and women will undergo FGM in this and coming years? Why isn't stopping this abuse an absolute priority, everywhere?

The commentaries, observations and narratives in this book are by more than 70 people from 27 countries, women and men who range in age from 13 to well beyond retirement — survivors, family members, campaigners and involved professionals. The stories explore aspects of FGM, which shed light both on how the practice remains a reality, imperilling the futures, even lives, of millions of women and girls around the world, and on what must be done to support survivors and relegate this harmful practice to history forever.

***

Imagine. You are a small girl, maybe ten years old, living in the bush somewhere sub-Saharan. It is early morning but already there are people milling everywhere in noisy celebratory mood.

Your mother rouses you and says, 'Today is The Day. Hurry! We must take you to the river to be cleansed in preparation. The herbalist will be here soon.'

Obediently, you follow your mother and other girls and some female relatives to the river, running cold after the night. Your clothes are removed, and you sit with your friends in the rushing water until your lower body is chilled.

Re-dressed in beautiful new attire, you return to the village, where family and neighbours are dancing and singing, fuelled by the potent local brew. There is a hut where something special going on. Instructed with your friends who also went to the river to join the queue, you wait to find out what is happening.

But the hut is dark, and within it all is not well. A girl is shrieking, women are singing too lustily. Alas, it is too late; your turn arrives and you enter uncertainly.

Your mother is suddenly nowhere to be seen. Three older women, one of them your own grandmother, strip off your lovely party clothes and force your legs apart …

You try to shout out, but someone gags you. The pain is intolerable as a woman goes about her business, cutting, scraping and stitching until you can no longer even writhe in protest. Betrayed by those you trusted most, beyond tears, too weak to move and shaking uncontrollably, you find your legs have been tied together, and you are carried to a makeshift bed to recuperate.

You dare not cry out again; the family's honour is at stake. Already bruised, perhaps even with fractured bones from being held down so tightly, passing urine will also require great courage for the next several days. It will feel as though your body is on fire.

And soon, you will be required to parade around your village with the other recently 'cut' girls, so that men may choose whom to purchase as a wife, perhaps as an extra bride to go alongside a more senior spouse. This financial transaction completed, your family will have reaped the benefit of the investment made in your brutal initiation all too soon to 'adult' status.

You will be at the disposal of your new husband, no longer the property of your father.

Very shortly you may discover you are pregnant, your young body still unready to carry a child.

Unlike your best friend (who was, you are told, possessed by bad spirits) you survived the genital mutilation recently inflicted. But will you survive the reopening on your wedding night? Will either you or your child survive pregnancy and birth? Afterwards, will you endure the unending nightmare of obstetric fistula?

In truth, no one knows, and very few, perhaps none, in your community perceive the links between your perils past and those still to come. These matters, they tell you, are determined by the gods or other ethereal forces. What will be will be.

How different your life will become from that of your cousin, who made it to safety in the refuge nearer town. She has managed to evade the 'cut' and is still in school.

While this particular story is fictional it is typical of the scenario faced by three million girls across the globe every year.

These girls' external genitals – their labia and clitoris – are cut, perhaps completely hacked away. In some instances, they are then sewn up so that almost nothing except a small opening is left where before they had healthy, well lubricated and elastic apertures for elimination, sex and giving birth.

FGM can happen almost anywhere. The notion that it is a custom 'only' to be found 'in Africa' is, as we shall see, seriously misinformed. The commentators who contributed to this book come from five different continents – and we know too that the missing one, South America, also has pockets at least of the practice, for instance in Colombia. There have also always been some 'medical' practices that equate to FGM in nations such as the United States and the United Kingdom, but with the growth of the diaspora, Western nations now also face a very serious challenge in eradicating FGM.

As one informant tells us, FGM is the most common form of child abuse in Britain.

In some communities around the world FGM is performed in the first few weeks of life. Most often, it occurs in mid-childhood, somewhere around the age of eight or ten, or it might occur just before (often very early) marriage or even whilst pregnant.

Worryingly however there is evidence that the age at which girls are mutilated is dropping – the perpetrators may suppose this is 'kinder'; and they don't want the child to recall or report the event.

Sometimes the mutilation is relatively superficial, in other instances it is a deeply invasive wound and much skin and flesh is carved away, before the remaining flesh is re-sutured to leave just a pinhole for the passing of urine and menstrual blood.

The damage may even be re-inflicted on a mother every time she has a baby.

To the great concern of the global medical community, clinically trained operatives, anaesthetic and sterile instruments are increasingly involved, ostensibly making it seem that the mutilation is modern and acceptable. Traditionally the 'cutting' is most often conducted on several children at once, at least until recently with shared 'instruments' – broken glass, a sharp stone, traditional knives, even fingernails – and without pain control or asepsis of any sort.

Whenever and however FGM occurs, it offers no health benefits whatsoever to the victim. It often causes lifelong medical problems, it is usually traumatising and it not infrequently results in death (either in the short-term or prematurely later in life, perhaps of both a mother and her newborn child).

Hearing the practice described in these ways, new enquirers are totally at a loss to understand why FGM occurs, or how it can have continued over literally millennia.

This book asks and seeks through the narrative of our many contributors to understand:

- What FGM comprises and how it varies
- Which peoples have undertaken FGM in the past, and which still do it now
- The rationales and beliefs which underlie the practices and
- The consequences of FGM, for the victim, for their communities, and for us all.

We will also learn a lot about communities, perhaps our own, where FGM has not traditionally been practised.

- Why are there increasing numbers of women and girls in Western countries who have had or are at risk of FGM?
- Are there laws against FGM? (The short answer here is, yes – in many nations around the world.)
- What is being done to stop FGM, in traditionally practising societies and in the 'West'?

And, most importantly of all, we will ask, what can we learn from those with direct experience of FGM who are seeking to eradicate it? And what can we do to help?

- What can victims – who often insist as adults that they are 'survivors', not 'victims'– tell us about FGM and how to confront it? What are their personal stories?
- How can those, sometimes survivors themselves, sometimes not, who lead the way in combating FGM help us to understand the challenges and opportunities ahead?
- What are the roles of policy makers, politicians and the media?
- And… what can we do ourselves, as concerned citizens wanting to make a better, healthier world for women, girls and their families everywhere?

All this, drawing on observations and ideas from many sources to examine what FGM means and how it can be stopped, is offered in the context of acknowledgement that those in modern Western countries – where traditionally FGM has not occurred – are not in a position to take an absolute position of moral superiority. We too (I speak for my own country, the United Kingdom) have much to be ashamed of.

Child abuse of various sorts continues to blight the lives of large numbers of defenceless children, inequalities of health and prospects are often huge, and patriarchy still rules in numerous ways to the detriment of many, men as well as women.

But in the end, none of these provisos changes the fundamental precepts which underpin this situation:

- FGM is amongst the most serious and cruel forms of human rights abuse.
- FGM often robs a woman of her sexuality, even before she is aware of it - she may never know much about sexual pleasure and love.
- FGM ruins health and sometimes kills.
- FGM can traumatise small children for the remainder of their lives.
- FGM is hugely damaging to entire economies.
- FGM is, in the most profound meaning of the word, an abomination.

It's estimated that FGM claims another victim somewhere in the world every ten or eleven seconds.

Understanding how this can happen is the key to making certain that, soon, it will never again blight lives to the shame of us all.

***

Some of those represented here are the amazing colleagues with whom I've been collaborating for a while. Some of them have been active with me on previous campaigns, and perhaps even advisers when I wrote my first book, *Eradicating Female Genital Mutilation: A UK Perspective* (Ashgate, 2015). But most of the people you will meet in this book I 'found' via Twitter and through other social media connections. For months I put out feelers across my social media interfaces, inviting anyone who might be interested to contact me for more information on this project.

It takes a long time to reach out across the globe on difficult issues such as FGM. I am enormously grateful to each of our contributors for responding, whether they were approached by me or they made contact themselves, agreeing to complete the questionnaire from which the information we now offer was extracted. Everyone who responded to my open invitation and shared their ideas and information is included in this book.

The format of the questionnaire, which I devised and piloted over several months is available on *Female Mutilation Worldwide*, the website which accompanies this book. My questions, along with innumerable individual, private email and telephone conversations, enabled me to construct a 'narrative' account for each respondent – for many of whom English is a second or simply foreign language.

In every case, I have done my level best to remain faithful to the information and ideas they have so generously shared, and wherever possible I have also re-checked with the person concerned, sometimes on several occasions, to try to be sure I have reflected their views and experience accurately. Omissions or misrepresentations may nonetheless sometimes remain. For these I apologise unreservedly, both to the person concerned and to the reader. I aim to correct any such inadvertent errors as soon as possible via the *Female Mutilation Worldwide* website.

With these caveats duly noted, our generous correspondents have taken us on an extraordinary journey.

We begin our travels with a close look at Kenya, the African country thought by many to have made the most overt advances in challenging FGM in a 'traditional, practising' context. The evidence and opinions offered here are illuminating and thought-provoking. It might be fair to say Kenya is at a crossroads in the fight to stop FGM, as various authorities and some citizens campaign vigorously against the ages-old customs and ways of traditional communities.

Next comes a journey, west to east, and then south, across the whole of Sub-Saharan and Southern Africa. Again, challenges and changes are emerging.

The following leg of our journey is from Northeast Africa (Egypt) via the Middle East to Southeast Asia, specifically, Indonesia. During this traverse it becomes evident that those tacking FGM must take on first the reluctance of many in authority to acknowledge that FGM is actually a problem. For much of this part of the world there is as yet barely a public vocabulary with which the concept of FGM can be examined, let alone a will proactively and officially to eradicate it. (The same deep reservations are true of some places in South America. We shall not visit that continent in the course of the present journey, but FGM also occurs there – as we noted for instance, in Colombia – although few are willing to acknowledge or discuss it.)

Australia is the stopping point after Indonesia. Here we have an opportunity to observe as a case study the emergence of a lobby (in which for clarity it must be noted I had some initial involvement) against FGM.

After Australia comes North America, mostly citizens of the United States, some originating from very different parts of the world, and a few Canadians. Here, in a different guise, observers might perceive the failure in some instances of public discourse to accommodate the vocabulary and realities of FGM, or even an inability to address publicly the practicalities of stopping abuse.

Crossing the Atlantic, we arrive next in Continental Europe. European nations north to south are included in our tour - here too we note the differences as well as the similarities of the challenges FGM presents in the various geographically dispersed elements of the diaspora. By now it must be evident to all who have shared our journey that there is no one, straightforward and obvious, way to make FGM history.

Finally we reach the United Kingdom, where significant efforts to end FGM have been made over the past few years.

As in previous chapters, a range of reports of case studies illustrates the complexities of the task with which campaigners in Britain are confronted. These reports illustrate how we must all respond as we can, drawing on whatever resources we can muster, to the challenge of eradicating the appalling practice of FGM forever.

Our global contributors to this book have generously shared a wide range of understandings of what FGM 'means' and how it should be addressed. The debates about how to eradicate FGM will continue for a while yet.. Whilst views on details may vary, however, the determination to spare future generations this cruel harm will without doubt continue unabated.

To return to the message with which we began this journey:

Female genital mutilation is everyone's business.

***

A note on chosen terminology in this book

For the removal of any doubt, I am a white, Western woman and feminist sociologist. There is no question in my own mind – the debate is examined in detail in my previous book - that female genital mutilation is just that: FGM is 'mutilation'.

Further, FGM must be positioned within a patriarchal conceptual framework. This belief was informed and bolstered by the *Bamako Declaration* (2005) and the earlier stated preference for the term FGM (1990) of the *Inter-African Committee on Traditional Practices Affecting the Health of Women and Children* (known as the IAC and led by Dr Kouyaté, author of the Preface to this book).

Deliberations such as *Bamako* and the IAC's position also led me and some of my campaigning colleagues, all with different experiences and from different perspectives, to produce the 2013 *Feminist Statement on Female Genital Mutilation.*

This current publication is, however, no place to impose my own choice of terminologies. I am profoundly grateful to all who took time and trouble to collaborate with me in developing the material which follows. I have of course, without reservation, respected each person's preferred terms as they share their narrative.

....

For references and weblinks, more information and further discussion of material and ideas in this book, please visit the Female Mutilation Worldwide website, at http:// femalemutilationworldwide.com.

CHAPTER 2:

What is Female Genital Mutilation?

Why is it 'mutilation'? Why does it happen? What is being done about it?

All female genital mutilation involves some sort of harm for non-medical reasons to the sexual organs of a girl, woman or even a female baby. It is easy to understand why the French amongst others call this damage female *sexual* mutilation.

Beyond the common theme of damage, however, there are many different ways in which this harm is inflicted.

The World Health Organisation (WHO), an organisation now existing for over half a century, has very serious concerns about FGM. It defines four main types of FGM:

1. Clitoridectomy: removal to whatever extent of the clitoris, an elongated, sensitive and erectile organ of which only a small part, the sensitive 'button' at the front is visible. It would be almost impossible to remove the entire clitoris, as it extends backwards in a wishbone shape around the vagina. Nor (because the victim usually moves, and the operator's skills may be minimal) is it normally possible to remove 'only' the prepuce, which is the fold of skin surrounding the visible clitoris.

2. Excision: removal of at least some of the clitoris, and also of the labia minora (the inside 'lips' which surround the vagina) plus, in some cases, the removal of the labia majora, the outside 'lips'.

3. Infibulation: when the labia, whether or not otherwise cut or scraped away, are sealed (often sewn, with pins, thread or thorns) so that only a small hole remains for the excretion of urine and menstrual blood. The clitoris is often excised before the infibulation, and the girl's legs may be bound together for some weeks to ensure the 'seal' is effectively formed.

4. Other: this may include piercing, scraping, cauterising (burning), pricking, lengthening or pulling the labia or otherwise harming the female genitalia.

FGM is often carried out by maternal grandmothers or aunts, or by traditional birth attendants (often called TBAs or 'midwives') or others, including sometimes men, with a position in the community who have no clinical training. Increasingly, however, especially amongst wealthier and / or better educated populations, it is done by people with modern medical skills.

It has been argued that so-called 'medicalisation' is 'better', because the act is more likely to be delivered hygienically and with pain control. There is some evidence, however, that medicalisation also results in a greater degree of excision. The World Health Organisation and many national medical bodies are very clear that, whatever the circumstances, no-one anywhere with clinical qualifications should be involved in this practice, and that to be party to FGM is a serious ethical and professional misdemeanour as well as, almost everywhere in the world, a crime.

The rationales for FGM vary across communities and belief sets, and across time. Whilst often the traducing of any particular 'reason' will be followed by a different one, amongst those commonly noted are that FGM:

- reduces sexual desire and enables young women to control their sexuality (which, it is believed, would otherwise be rampant),
- increases modesty and purity (required by various religions and belief sets) and keeps the girl 'clean',
- increases bride price or dowry for the family and the likelihood of a 'good' marriage(essential for the parents in old age, as their 'pension'). These 'marriages' are often however contracted (by fathers and 'husbands') when girls are still at an age when sexual intercourse would be perceived by external observers as child rape – and the man may already have other wives,
- keeps the wife faithful – both for fear of pain if, in the course of illicit passion, she is deinfibulated, and because the deinfibulation will be evident, and punished,
- removes the perceived risk – a 'belief trap' which no-one dare test – of death which would arise if a man's penis, or a newborn child's head, were to touch the clitoris (which is sometimes believed to continue to grow, as a 'third leg', if not removed),
- is an important element of maintaining traditions and customs, sometimes required also by religion and
- may be (re)introduced where before it did not previously occur, either to fit in after a group moves to a new community, or else to define the group (diaspora) as different from its host society.

Despite these and many other claimed rationales for FGM, in reality it inflicts only harm. If it is not done, the harm will not arise. There are no 'benefits' beyond the increase, where such is the currency, in prospects for marriage and bride price.

Essentially, FGM confirms girls and women as simply economic commodities invested in by men (but often processed on their behalf by women) for other men. Tragically this investment, whilst bringing some economic return for the investor in the shorter term, has but limited longer term real return or reward for any party. It also often triggers lifelong ill-health and disability for the 'commodity' herself.

Nonetheless, even the fatalities – sometimes in large numbers, perhaps even 10 per cent or more in some locations, that follow FGM are explained away. It was fate, or bad spirits, community leaders will say, not the 'cutting', which caused the girls' deaths.

And for every death, there are many other victims of FGM whose lives are never again the same.

The immediate physical risks are obvious, ranging from haemorrhage, shock, tetanus and rampant infections, to broken bones (from the struggle of being held down) and damaged organs. Later, there may be recurrent urinary infections, open sores, a higher risk of HIV, cysts and many other persistently unpleasant and painful conditions.

Then there are the deep psychological wounds. Whether she is persuaded to 'volunteer' or is harshly kidnapped, the child undergoing FGM has been betrayed, her trust destroyed, by some or all of the people she holds most dear. No-one was there to protect her at her hour of greatest need.

It is not surprising that some women with FGM say the psychological, sometimes psychiatric, issues which arise post-event are even harder to bear than the physical ones. For some, too, it may be unsurprising that they choose in years to come to revisit the harm on their own daughters. They cannot countenance any thought that their mothers permitted FGM to be performed on them without compelling reason.

Also, sometimes far too soon after FGM has been inflicted, there are the risks associated with pregnancy and childbirth. Conception itself may be difficult, labour may be constricted, obstetric fistula (permanent tearing between the vagina and the bladder or rectum) may occur with truly horrendous life-long outcomes, and the child, male or female, may die or suffer permanent damage because of the difficult delivery. Even children who survive delivery are at extra risk, as women with FGM have a considerably higher overall maternal mortality of those without it. In Sub-Saharan Africa many children are tragically left motherless each year. These children are ten times more likely than others to die within two years of their mothers' deaths.

In short, as a contributor to this book reminds us, female genital mutilation is truly the 'gift' that keeps on giving; or, perhaps even more grimly, that keeps on taking.

At long last the nations of the world are starting to acknowledge the dimensions of this gendered global pandemic – to reiterate, WHO believes about 130+ million women and girls are living with FGM, and another three million undergo it every year – and the global community is responding more definitively to the crisis.

Since 2003, there has been an annual *International Day of Zero Tolerance to FGM*, observed on 6 February. The day was that year by Stella Obasanjo, then First Lady of Nigeria, who declared it so during a conference organised by the *Inter-African Committee of Traditional Practices Affecting the Health of Women and Children* (the IAC), and is now observed by the United Nations to mark the struggle to make the practice history for all time.

Almost a decade later, very importantly, in 2012 the United Nations General Assembly adopted a resolution on the elimination of FGM; and before that, in 2010, the WHO and UN partner organisations published a global strategy to stop the medicalisation of FGM.

Since that time, in 2013, the United Nations Children's Fund (UNICEF) has published a 'statistical overview and exploration of the dynamics of change'. This publication offers analysis, drawing on seventy nationally representative surveys over a 20-year period, of trends and the relative success of various approaches in eliminating FGM in 29 African and Asian countries where FGM was then known to occur. This, the most authoritative global report on FGM ever, concluded that progress in eradication was being made, patchily and painfully slowly.

More recently still, in 2014 and 2015 Ban Ki-moon, the Secretary General of the United Nations, has been overt in his robust condemnation of and focus on FGM, working actively with campaigners world-wide, and with *The Guardian* to deliver a real step change and momentum in efforts to eradicate it.

It seems that, though often far too lethargically, we as the global community are learning more about, and acknowledging, where and why FGM occurs, and how the many valiant efforts in pockets around the globe – some of them evidenced in this book - can be conjoined to greater effect.

What now needs to be done is, in some respects at least, straightforward – more education, greater legal vigilance, better health care and more opportunities for women outside domestic servitude, in every community affected.

Other aspects require a more nuanced approach. The influencing variables are multitude. In practising communities the mindsets of the group leaders (or sometimes brutal regulators) are critical; but so perhaps are the modes of thought of those seeking to change minds on a more global scale. How, fundamentally, are we to understand and respond to FGM?

At what point, for example, do we as campaigners and professionals who seek to combat FGM, turn from accepting and accommodating terminologies to the much starker language of human rights and entitlement?

When and how does reference to 'cutting' and 'female circumcision' become, quite bluntly, the truth, that FGM is 'genital mutilation'? Why do some campaigners still insist on euphemism? Why do some people demand that Westerners allow cultural relativism – that is, 'respect' for a different set of values - in regard to FGM, usually performed on black girls in communities with non-Western traditions, than we would for white children in Western society? At what point should or do the harsh realities of legal sanction, including prison, take over from sweet words of 'respect', or reason and persuasion?

These and many other questions are posed vividly, and answered in striking and contrasting ways, by the resolute contributors to this volume.

For further, more formal reportage and consideration of these issues, readers may wish to refer to this author's detailed textbook, *Eradicating Female Genital Mutilation* (Ashgate, 2015). The current book, however, provides a multitude of real stories about real people across the globe who have chosen to confront FGM in their own lives.

Doubtless we all begin our 'global journey' here with a number of more or less confirmed views about female genital mutilation. It is probable that some of the contributions in the pages that follow will challenge those views. Nor, when we complete our travels, will we have been reassured by any overall consensus on every issue about how to respond to what we have seen.

The 'vocabulary of FGM' is currently far from universal. There is a long way to go before we can speak with one shared voice on all these matters; but that is one reason why the diverse perspectives of our contributors are so important.

On one point, however, there is unequivocal concurrence. Female genital mutilation must stop. Now.

The issues around FGM are complex and constantly changing. Consideration of these changes and questions and news about progress in combating FGM can be found on the Female Mutilation Worldwide website, which also provides weblinks and other further reading. Readers are warmly welcome to engage in these discussions. Now, however, having reviewed a stereotypical account of what in practice female genital mutilation involves, we will turn, in the chapters which follow, to reports from people who have themselves experienced or observed FGM at first hand.

These first-hand accounts will not be easy reading, but they will help us to understand this harmful traditional practice better. Learning more about the horrors of FGM will help us to move towards hope for an FGM-free world in the future.

CHAPTER 3:

Kenya

Nearly, but not quite all, countries in the world, including Kenya, have made FGM illegal. In 2012 a United Nations declaration voted unanimously, in a proposal put forward by the nations of the Africa Group, to take all necessary steps to end FGM.

Our contributors from Kenya illustrate how much this nation is in many ways taking a lead in respect to the fight against female genital mutilation. The harm about which FGM survivors speak here is unimaginable to those who have not endured it; but these survivors must be heard. Increasingly, these resolute women campaigners are being joined by others (some of them active escapees from the knife). All of them determined, with their steadfast male compatriots and supporters from other parts of the world, that current and future generations of girls will remain intact.

In Kenya about 50 per cent of women have undergone FGM. This country is, however, amongst those traditionally practising nations where significant progress is now being made in eradicating the practice. It is helpful therefore that alongside contributions from community and voluntary organisations we have commentary from the Head the Prosecution Unit on FGM in the Office of the Kenyan Director of Public Prosecutions. We need to understand the damage FGM inflicts on individuals and communities, but we must also appreciate the steps that countries like Kenya are taking to make this horrifying abuse history.

THE SURVIVORS

The women who report their genital mutilation here reflect a wide range of experience. Ann Njambi struggles in the slums of Nairobi against ill-health, HIV and poverty, whilst also helping the charity Compassion, a community based organisation (CBO), to refute FGM. Virginia Mukwanyagah Gibson also supports Compassion CBO, and Judy Kerubo is a young teacher educating mothers about FGM.

Jackline, still a young schoolgirl in the Rift Valley area of Kenya, experienced FGM as a pre-teen, and now counters the practice amongst her friends. Severina

Lemachokoti is a teacher and counselling psychologist who founded the Naretu Girls and Women Empowerment Programme in Samburu County. Asha Ismail is a Kenyan who founded a charity, Save A Girl, Save A Generation in Spain, and campaigns both there and in the Kenyan Somali community.

Other Kenyan survivors include Lucy Mashua Sharp who now campaigns in the USA and Valentine Nkoyo, also from the Maasai community, who now lives and campaigns in Britain.

Ann Njambi

I underwent female genital mutilation in 1985, at the age of 15. I live in my hometown, Kiambu, Central Province, where it is our culture for girls to undergo FGM. I belong to the Kikuyu community, which is among those who practice FGM. Other practicing communities include the Embu, Meru and Tharaka.

My parents took me to have FGM, and we were accompanied by other women and girls. Everyone was involved: my parents, my clan and the woman who did the procedure.

The circumciser used one knife to cut all of us. This was the knife that was used for all the village girls for years. I remember it was not sterilised and we went in turn. Afterwards I stayed in bed for a whole month and I bled a lot. It was done without anaesthesia.

FGM is accompanied by bleeding and infection. You can spend a month on a sick bed, sharing first the knife, and then the towel, bed and sheets.

It was a terrible, harrowing experience, very painful, with a scar that never heals.

There is no discussion about what happened after you are cut. It is something no one wants to talk about. You are simply told you are now mature – no longer a girl – and you are given a woman to care for you and help you during the healing process. She is in charge of washing you and teaching you the traditional ways, and telling you how you should now behave.

Unfortunately I acquired a longstanding infection in the FGM wound. Because of my wound, when I got married the man later divorced me.

The man also infected me with HIV/AIDS.

All this has affected me psychologically as well as physically. I feel betrayed and as though I am not complete. It is like being an amputee of any other part of the body.

FGM is a torture of unimaginable magnitude. You feel guilty. You have low esteem.

Now I work with a voluntary organisation, Compassion CBO, to stop FGM. The only way to eradicate it is to work at grassroots level and, via seminars, to get members of the public educated to cease practising it. Speaking against FGM is still perceived as speaking against our community.

So, even now, FGM continues; but what has changed is the knife. No longer is there any sharing, and today FGM is done not by traditional midwives, but secretly, by medics.

Traditional practising communities keep supporting FGM. They cannot be trusted to stop. For FGM to end, mainstream society must become involved.

Society must come up with laws to criminalise FGM. Others can help by organizing forums where we are invited to air our views.

***

Virginia Mukwanyagah Gibson

I was 'initiated' in 1987 in my father's house in Maara Tharaka Nithi County so I experienced female genital mutilation directly. It is our tradition for girls to undergo FGM at the age of puberty or beyond; I was 11 years old when I underwent FGM. My mother accompanied me to the ceremony where other girls of my age also joined me. It was a very painful operation. The initiator used one blunt knife to cut all 12 of us in turn. The knife was unsterilised. The experience was very painful and tormenting, something which one would be eager to forget.

Note that I had asked to undergo FGM. Remember that it is illegal to perform FGM in our county.

The clan and my parents were very involved; the circumciser does it at their request. After I was initiated I was taken to seclusion in a room in my mother's house where I lay on my back in bed for almost a month. I bled a lot but I eventually healed, leaving a big scar on my vagina.

During the healing period I had a special woman who was my chaperone, who washed me daily and mentored me. As I was now a mature girl, having undergone the circumcision, this woman taught and advised me how I should conduct myself once I was again out in the community.

At first I felt honoured and happy that I had been initiated, but then I married and I did not enjoy sex, due to the painful scar – though I did not want my husband to notice.

My first-born child arrived five years later, when I was 16. The experience was terrible. The scar started to bleed due to muscle stress during labour; but I soldiered on to become the proud mother of four children.

Psychologically, FGM affects me due to low sexual satisfaction, and my husband is also affected. We live in pretence whenever possible; I prefer to forget about that for my peace of mind.

FGM continues. It is still practiced mainly in secret by midwives and doctors. The knives are not shared and they are sterilised and healing is medically cared for. Remember there is a general belief that FGM controls sexual urges and libido in girls. It's thought to reduce illicit sex in unmarried girls. To some extent uncircumcised girls may find it difficult to get a suitor; and there are also other harmful traditional practices such as marrying off underage girls after FGM.

I belong to the Meru community, which is far away from eradicating FGM. It's culturally cherished by the Meru and other communities such as the Embu, Kikuyu, Tharaka, Kisii and Mbere. It is difficult to speak out against FGM in these communities. You are easily pointed out if you challenge their traditions, which they hold very important.

I believe FGM can be eradicated, through seminars and workshops where the public is generally taught and educated on the dangers of FGM. Community leaders and politicians should be the first to endorse these teachings.

Mainstream society must be involved in stopping FGM. Traditionally involved communities cannot do it alone.

***

Judy Kerubo

I work for a women's organisation in Kisii Nyanza province, Kenya, where I was born.

I underwent female genital mutilation at our rural home more than a decade ago, at the age of 12. Once the wound was healed life just went on as normal. I haven't seen the people who did it again since that day.

I haven't as yet been blessed with a family, and now I have a job in a women's organisation in Agape, as a teacher. I would like to teach young mothers to stop FGM, and tell them about the disadvantages, so they will stop subjecting their daughters to it.

It bothers me when people say a woman who underwent FGM is in even greater pain when giving birth than a woman who has not undergone FGM.

We must teach the women who circumcise these girls, and tell them about the disadvantages of FGM and the advantages of not practicing it. Communities still insist it's their culture and say therefore they cannot stop it, so society as a whole must become involved in preventing FGM.

My message to decision makers in Kenya is simple: jail those who still do those things.

***

Jackline

I am a student at the Lenkai Christian School in Kimana, in the Rift Valley of Kenya, and I campaign against female genital mutilation, which I was forced to experience last year, when I was 12.

I was living with my parents in Rombo Loitokitok, a sub-county in Kenya. That was when father told me that I was to undergo the FGM and then get married to an old man. I couldn't argue or say anything because in my culture men are the decision makers.

On the day of the cut I recall there was an old lady, my mother, an aunt and neighbours who really support FGM. I bled nearly to death and afterwards my mum helped me to escape and I couldn't walk, but she had no alternative about the FGM.

One month later, when I had recovered from the FGM, I was cheated and deceived. They said I was going to visit my aunt, but I found out that I had already been married off.

I escaped by walking 15 kilometres to find Mr. Leshinga, who advocates for ending FGM within my community. He took me to the chief, then the following day I was taken in by Mrs. Dorcus Parit, who rescued me and gave me a place to call home.

I am now 13 years old, an activist and survivor of FGM. I have decided to be in the lead in activism to end FGM in my school and community. It has been a challenge, I feel stigmatised whenever I go to shower with other girls and they see I am different from them.

FGM is very common in the Maasai community and I am afraid many of us young girls are undergoing it. In the Maasai community ladies are seen as objects. They are not allowed to speak out loud over the FGM issues, or talk in front of men.

I am involved in advocacy and in a mentoring programme with girls to end FGM. I go to schools, outreaching to both primary and secondary schoolchildren, sharing my stories to educate young girls and support them. I tell them what happened to me and that I would like them to make sound decisions and to be against FGM.

Everyone in my new community is involved in supporting advocacy to end FGM, which leads to early marriages. In my culture after the cut we are told that we are now old enough to have our own family and this contributes to high dropout rates of girls in schools around Loitokitok.

For us to be successful I would request other stakeholders and the government of Kenya to support us in activism to end FGM in the Maasai community.

***

Severina Lemachokoti

I am a mother of two, a trained teacher and a counselling psychologist. I am also a survivor of female genital mutilation and founder of a community based organisation, the Naretu Girls and Women Empowerment Programme, which works to sensitise the community on the harmful cultural practices that affect the girls and women socially, physically and psychologically.

My community is in Samburu County, Northern Kenya, where we are bound by cultural practices that affect girls and women. One of these harmful traditional practices is female genital mutilation, to which I was subjected as a child.

Other examples of these cultural practices include early and forced marriages, beading (where young girls are 'engaged' to young warriors, the Morans) and traditional abortion (a brutal practice which can follow from the beading).

FGM is one of the worse practices and I do a lot of training country wide with the support of other NGOs like AMREF, World Vision, Fida Kenya, Compassion International and the Ministry of Health.

In the Kenyan Constitution FGM is prohibited, to protect the girl child. The government made a step to constitute anti-FGM boards to help in implementing the law especially in the counties that practice FGM.

The politicians fear to talk about FGM to the people since they fear to lose votes during elections. They prefer to keep quiet, rather than talking about it.

This silence has given us problems in trying to convince the communities to abandon FGM, in line with our constitution.

Our administration officers at the village level (most of them are illiterate) are afraid to arrest or report cases of FGM; they fear the community. Just a few months ago, men from my community had a very big meeting at which they declared FGM a cultural practice that should be continued … unless the government comes out clearly to tell them why the practice needs to be abandoned!

We may gather from this that a lot of education and sensitisation is needed for our men to change and support the campaign.

I am a survivor of FGM and I got my education through a missionary scholarship. I am basically giving back to my community, whose illiteracy rate is 70 per cent.

***

Asha Ismail

It's been 41 years, but the sound of the blade still rings in my head.

We lived in a border town between Kenya and Ethiopia. I was just a small child when my mother sent me to buy the razor blades for the great day of my so-called 'purification'.

I was happy because I thought that it would be something nice. I thought that my life would change for the better. I was five years old.

But what awaited me was very far from beautiful. It was a nightmare, one that I have never woken up from.

At the beginning, I did not understand what was going to happen. I was with my mom, and waiting for me in my grandmother's kitchen were my grandmother (may she rest in peace) and another old woman whom I had never met before. The kitchen had mud walls and floor and a thatched roof, like all the rest of the rooms in my grandmother's compound.

The women had made a hole in a corner of the kitchen and covered it with an old sack; that was my operating room. My grandmother was seated on the floor with her legs wide spread and they asked me to remove my underwear and lift up my little dress, then I was made to sit.

I resisted just a little bit and my grandmother forced my legs open with her own. And there, without any sanitary assistance or any type of anaesthesia, the old lady mutilated me for the rest of my life!

They stripped off my clitoris, cut my labia minora and majora, and then stitched everything together, sealing me. They used a needle and a thread. Like a piece of cloth I was stitched.

Much later in life I came to learn that what they did to me was one of the worst of the four types of FGM that are practiced: infibulation. They left me a hole the size of a match for my bodily needs.

The pain I felt was so intense that even today I cannot describe it. I tried to scream with all my strength, but I couldn't because they had put a rag in my mouth. According to my family it was shameful to hear the screaming – a woman should not show her pain they told me.

Finally, I got healed, or so I thought. What I did not know was that my nightmare had only just begun. I could go on... it's permanent damage, it's a mutilation. I always insist female genital *mutilation* is the perfect description of what was done to us.

Today I cannot sew a button. I am unable to see a needle.

The most horrific part was however still to come. I had to spend a month sitting and tied from the toes to the waist so that the infibulation would close and seal properly. I could only pee out droplets, and the pain was terrible. Why did my mother do this to me? I wondered.

But 40 years ago it was just part of life. No questions were asked and no accusations made. My mother was simply fulfilling her duty, which was to ensure that I came to marriage as a virgin. Only this way could *she* walk with her head high among her people.

Apparently, my mother later recalled, I told her that if I ever got a daughter I will never permit this to happen to her. And yes, I questioned my mother and asked other girls during all my childhood and teenage life, about why this was done to us, but no one wanted to discuss the topic.

So I am an FGM survivor and an activist, though it took time for my family to realise that I was serious. But they have finally accepted me, and they support me. I am single. I have divorced twice, and I have three children, a girl and two boys, but I just don't seem to cope with men. I am before anything a proud mother of three, with a high level of education in Kenya.

My daughter is the first saved generation and the major reason for my decision to take action. She is 25 years old. I started my fight against a FGM when my daughter was born.

It's common knowledge that many women, and particularly African women, go through untold suffering in their lives, and more so when pregnant, during delivery, when rearing their children and during calamities such as draught, floods, wars and politically or ethnically motivated, or resource based, conflicts. They are subjected to more than they can bear.

I have founded an organisation called *Save A Girl, Save A Generation*. We work in Kenya, where we have a small group of three or four volunteers based in Garissa, town and county who focus on affected children there, mostly in the Somali community. A high percentage of the residents (90 per cent) practise FGM as culturally inherited tradition, so the eradication of FGM is an urgent need.

But these days I usually live in Spain. The Spanish arm of my charity comprises a group of five women who had one goal in common, to save the girls. *Save A Girl, Save A Generation* has been registered in Spain since 2007, although we have been working together quietly for the past twenty years. We have never been funded.

We saw the need to create awareness of female genital mutilation and other harmful traditions in Spain because of the increasing number of refugees from Somalia, Sudan and Ethiopia, among other countries where these practices are common. *Save A Girl, Save A Generation* is now a Spanish based nongovernmental organisation involved in addressing the problems of females as members of society from the East African region.

Women are married into a harem, some with co-wives older than their own mother, none screened for sexually transmittable diseases.

The girl child is seen as more of a liability, in contrast to boys. They are often not sent to schools or, if sent, not beyond primary level, from where they are seen to be ripe for marriage.

Unfortunately, we have found that the FGM fight is not giving as good results as expected, so we are studying also what is going wrong – a subject about which personally I have my own opinions.

More must be done by the authorities in Spain, too. In Spain the victims do not have any support and, although there are laws, the expertise of campaigners and survivors is not utilised.

And now things are becoming very difficult. FGM is being used to protest against the Western world, and there are other abuses too: early marriage, child prostitution, child labour and gender violence. All of society must be active against these abuses.

Education is a good weapon in the fight against FGM, teaching from primary level about how harmful it is. Introducing issues like bad and good traditions in schools at primary level can help to protect girls now, or, if they are victims already, this can help them save their daughters in the future.

A free telephone, with the support of the government for girls who want to save themselves from FGM, and protected accommodation (refuge) plus a trained, prepared reconciliation team can help in not separating families but uniting them once the danger is over.

I also believe that, although it's imposed on us to somehow please our so-called husbands and the community, women themselves can decide to put a stop to FGM. Women have an incredible strength when it comes to what they strongly believe in and when it comes to protecting their children. They can do miracles once they make up their mind. We just need to help women to realise they are strong and are able to choose not to mutilate.

More often FGM has been a taboo issue, always they disregard the matter.

FGM is the worst form of violation of human rights and gender abuse, and the world must unite to say 'Enough'.

....

OTHER WOMEN CAMPAIGNERS

Kenya has many different people campaigning against female genital mutilation, some of them survivors as above, but also others who have seen the devastation FGM can cause.

Four other Kenyan women, all still living in Kenya, and all seeking actively to erase the practice of FGM there, are Charity Waithera, an 18 year old volunteer for the Compassion CBO organisation, Domtila Chesang, now a teacher and a campaigner in Kenya with *The Guardian* newspaper, who as a child witnessed the brutality of the FGM ordeal and swore to avoid it for herself, Lucy Espila, who works as a Gender and Communications Officer for the development arm of the Catholic Church in Samburu, and Selestine Otom, who, with an MBA in Gender and Development, is Founder and Chief Executive of a women's rights NGO focussed on the prevention of gender-based violence (often referred to as GBV) and FGM.

Esther Oenga, who was born in Kenya, now lives in the UK, where she conducts research and campaigns against FGM. In Chapter 9 she offers a brief summary of the situation in Kenya and of her work in the UK.

***

Charity Waithera

I learned about female genital mutilation from my grandmother, who told me that it was conducted in an open field where boys and girls attended together. There was a specialist 'cutter' and then a ceremony.

My grandmother told me that every girl had to go through FGM because it was a mark of identity, and a sign of the transition from childhood to adulthood.

According to my granny's information, people from the community acted as witnesses, aunts were in attendance to mentor the girls, and the specialist initiated ('cut') them.

After the ceremony the initiates were taken to rooms by their given mentor, who guided and instructed the girls on how on how to take on their new responsibilities as adults. Nothing else happened afterwards.

I am now 18 years old and I am single. I have no family of my own. I would like to become involved in organisations against violation of girl child rights, and myself to get a mentor from such an organisation, a person who will always guide me as I proceed to the university.

I don't as yet have much idea on how to get involved with those people or organisations fighting FGM and other violations of girls' right, but I would like to learn how to take on the responsibilities of organising groups and educating people on dangers faced during FGM.

Violations of girls' rights affect my everyday life, because when I hear about cases of FGM, I think about how painful it is, and about the consequences it can have, such as death due to severe bleeding. I just wish it would come to an end.

We need more support, and sponsors, so that we can educate more people about the serious risks of the practice. Also, the people who still practise FGM – the Pokot, Samburu and Nandi communities – must be restrained, maybe by locking them in jail and fining them huge charges.

FGM is becoming less common in my community because of the introduction of education to both old and young generations, and people are becoming aware of the side effects and rights of the child, especially the girl child.

It remains difficult for people to speak out against these practices, because they still believe that everyone has to undergo FGM to be accepted in the community.

The authorities should be stricter on those who practise FGM or harm girls in other ways, such as the Maasai Community, who still permit early and forced marriages with young girls.

***

Domtila Chesang

I always knew about female genital mutilation because as a child I attended most of the local FGM ceremonies. I am a member of the Pokot community, one of the 42 tribes in Kenya. I am the second born in a family of six. I grew up with a very harsh background. My dad was very abusive and he abandoned us completely when I was ten.

The FGM 'ceremonies' (as they are called) were accompanied by a lot of feasting, but I had never thought of it as a cultural practice found only in my tribe and a few other tribes in my country. I assumed it something all human beings had to undergo.

FGM is performed by an old woman, an expert in the practice, usually on girls aged 12–17. It was not until my own cousin had it done, aged about 15, that I fully realised what FGM entails.

The Pokot community practises Type 3 FGM with no sewing, but the girls' legs are tied together for about a month so their wounds close up leaving a tiny hole. The FGM is done in two stages. The first stage is cutting off the clitoris, which is done in public, so I was aware of that, as were the other young girls.

Little did we know there was another second cutting, which is stage two. The girls are taken to the bush, leaves are spread on the ground for them to lie flat on their backs, naked, and older women pin them down singing loudly to cut out their screams.

Following my cousin, I sneaked to see what happened after the public ceremony. For the second stage only older women were permitted, but they didn't notice me because they were drunk. I saw it all. My cousin was lying down, screaming but helpless. She was overpowered by the women and all her genitals were cut out, so finally what was left was flat, red flesh.

A little later they bound my cousin's legs closed, and eventually, when she had healed, there was just a tiny hole left for urination and menstruation and to have sex and give birth.

My cousin was actually my saviour because after I witnessed her being butchered I decided to rebel; I went out to find why it is done, but when I asked my mother to explain FGM that same evening I found she had been silenced by the cut herself, and she didn't give me any answer. I later came to know that my cousin was married off immediately she after had healed, and that no other words were spoken about her, end of the story.

I got no satisfaction, so I ran away to a boarding school, still with the aim of starting a discussion on FGM. I stood my ground and refused to be cut, although I wasn't forced to have it by my mum.

And now I am an anti-FGM activist. In 2011 with my colleague Cath Holland from the UK, I helped to create the organisation, Kepsteno Rotwo Tipin ('Stop the Knife'), for which I remained a volunteer. I have helped organise Alternative Rites of Passage ceremonies (which we call ARPs), and workshops and seminars to train people young and old in my community about the effects of FGM.

I have also educated my extended family and immediate neighbours to abandon FGM. Personally, I helped influence my friends to refuse the cut with me when I rebelled. I am looking forward to working together in this fight with some of the most influential people in this world, especially ladies such as the film actor Angelina Jolie and the first lady of my country, Margaret Gakuo Kenyatta, who is especially concerned about maternal mortality and in 2014 was named UN Person of the Year. We have had a lot of support from *The Guardian* in collaborating with these global influencers.

I am currently active as volunteer Project Manager for Kepsteno Rotwo Tipin, training adolescent girls at risk of FGM. On the final day of our workshops we perform Alternative Rites of Passage ceremonies (ARPs) with parents and members of the community present to witness and accept the young girls into the adult community.

As a campaigner I am heavily affected by this practice. It is part of my day-to-day concern and has become my responsibility to eradicate it; I have had no peace ever since I got involved in these campaigns.

The Pokot and neighbouring communities have been practising FGM for generations, but it is becoming less common. A few years ago FGM was normally accompanied by public ceremonies but it is now carried out secretly. People know FGM is illegal so they do it in secret to avoid the long arm of the government.

Training and education for village elders in our communities will help a great deal since they are the decision makers who will bring even secret FGM to a halt.

It is still sometimes hard to speak out, especially when you are a woman – and worse, a young woman like myself - because in my community women are not valued. They are seen as vessels for giving birth, that is all. Not much else is expected from them.

Some people cut and marry off young girls just to acquire the cows, without caring what would become of the girls' lives and futures. This issue must be addressed by considering with the parents what they trade their daughters for.

In my view FGM should not be termed a cultural practice. Why would anyone 'correct' how your body is made in the name of 'culture'?

My message, not only to decision makers in my country but to the entire world and all women and leaders out there, is: Please, women have suffered enough. It's time to bring to an end this harmful oppressive practice.

FGM is a painful, oppressive, non-profitable, useless, harmful and barbaric practice.

***

Lucy Espila

I work as the Gender and Communications officer for Caritas Maralal, the development arm of the Catholic Church in Samburu County, Northwest Kenya.

Previously I had heard about Female Genital Mutilation in school, but I really didn't know how rampant it was till I got a job about two years ago at Caritas Maralal (with which Sayydah Garrett, is also involved). We received funding from CAFOD (Catholic Aid For Overseas Development) to mainstream gender in all our development projects. Our partners are World Vision, the Ministry of Gender and Social Services, Caritas Kenya, CAFOD and the Pastoralist Child Foundation.

One of the activities in our project is to train the communities on gender-based violence. Through engaging the communities we work with, researching a lot on this particular subject, and also listening to the facilitator, I learnt about FGM. I am 27, I haven't undergone FGM and I don't have a family of my own, but my gender work is important to me. I know that something has to be done to fight this endemic social vice.

In Samburu County female genital mutilation is a compulsory cultural practice on victims, who are brainwashed to believe it is an important rite of passage into womanhood.

I am among the key people involved in anti -FGM campaigns in Samburu County. This is done through facilitating awareness creation about this harmful cultural practice. The work is quite sensitive because the communities see you as a person who is out to question their culture, and FGM is a practice seen as important in the Samburu culture.

A different approach has to be used. My discussions with men from Samburu County give me mixed feelings. Some say 'we have to end this thing', others say 'you people have a long way to go... we can't end this'.

FGM can effectively be fought if the people of Samburu actually own these initiatives. Those working to end it should just support and empower the communities themselves to campaign against it. Otherwise people will attend workshops and go back home still willing to hold on to this harmful traditional practice.

The vicious cycle of this type of violence needs to be broken. It starts from the village elders, the circumcisers, the grand parents of the girl child, the parents of the girl child, the relatives, the community around her, the politicians who might be scared to be seen as people who are going against their culture, her prospective husband and the girl child herself.

I know various activists in Samburu County are doing their best to fight this vice. I have attended a variety of stakeholders meetings to discuss our interventions. What everyone points out is that there is a disconnect between the ideas and the reality.

Activities such as the 'Alternative Rites of Passage' (ARPs) have had their fair share of criticism from the communities and campaigners. Some ask 'What is the alternative?

Our girls will graduate under the "alternative rites of passage project" and still undergo FGM as well.'

We are also glad that the Anti-FGM Board in Kenya have now appointed an Anti-FGM coordinator in Samburu County. Mainstream society should be actively involved but the traditionally practicing communities should take the lead. That way the perception that people are out to use / attract 'donor money" to fight FGM can fade to the background.

In 2013, we held a training session on gender-based violence in Opiroi. This community in Samburu Central is still deeply rooted in retrogressive harmful cultural practices which have adversely affected development where women and the girl child are concerned. From our discussion with the workshop participants we learned that if a lady cheats on her husband and gives birth to a baby boy, the boy is killed. These are harmful traditional practices that must be stopped.

The problems are many. Girls get married at the age of 12, having undergone FGM. A clinical officer at Maralal District Hospital tells us that they admit cases of GBV on a weekly basis. He added that 19 cases of assault were admitted in August 2013. HIV/AIDS is a further concern.

We know that the county government of Pokot in Kenya allocated some funds to fight FGM, and this should also be the way forward also in Samburu County. The two levels of government should take the lead and partner with activists to develop a contingency plan. We need to end FGM in a conflict-sensitive way which still respects the beautiful culture of the Samburu people.

I want to see victims of gender-based violence being empowered to speak out ... and everyone working together to fight gender based violence.

***

Selestine Otom

I came to know about female genital mutilation through my work as the founder and chief executive of *Usalama*, a women's rights NGO which is concerned with gender based violence prevention and response in Kenya. I saw FGM being performed during a fact-finding mission in one region of Kenya.

A teenaged girl was being 'cut' (mutilated) by an elderly woman in the village. The mission programme sponsor recorded a video and did not leave us with a copy. I have never gone back to the village. Witnessing the actual cut happening to the young girl left me traumatised. Her screams and sobs during the cut were very scary.

The entire team that witnessed the FGM episode were taken for a debriefing session by a counsellor.

From then on we started mobilizing communities against FGM, and lobbying with lawmakers to draft an anti-FGM bill. That was later done and passed into law in 2011.

I am married with a family (three teenage children and five orphans and vulnerable children). The important people in my life are my family members, work mates and my women's rights' programme beneficiaries, but FGM does bother me in my line of work.

Maternal mortality rates are presumably higher in communities that practice FGM due to the fact that many girls get married off very soon after FGM, when their reproductive systems are unready to hold a baby for nine months. At times it's the mother, the baby or both loosing lives due to excess haemorrhage, or else it's prolonged labour leading to obstetric fistula.

Also, some young girls have acquired HIV during the cut, which is very sad and distressing indeed.

Working with men from early ages (teenage) is especially important, to instil into their heads that FGM must not happen, and ensure they do not discriminate against women who have not been mutilated when they choose a wife.

FGM is a sexual offence and a violation of human rights and everyone *must stop it*, and be involved in campaigning against it. It touches a lot on sexual reproductive health, including women's sexual rights.

Speaking about FGM is not easy in almost all communities that practise it because of the sacred nature of sexual matters in my country and many other African contexts. For some, sex topics are still perceived as taboo.

Community opinion leaders and decision makers, as well as elders, are best placed to champion the campaign against FGM, and to instil behavioural change among their followers.

My clear and precise message to decision makers in my country is to implement actively the Kenya Sexual Offences Act, 2006 which stipulates all categories of sex crimes, the penalties for the offenders and rehabilitation mechanisms for the survivors. Having that law on sexual offences is one thing. Making it work is another. It all depends on political good will.

Unfortunately, the national budgetary allocations to reproductive health services and activities is just a very small percentage of the Kenyan National Health budget, below 15 percent of the National Budget and therefore contrary to (less than) the Abuja Declaration to which signatory member States agreed.

This is a challenge, especially as most reproductive health programmes (advocacy, campaigns, and activities) are left largely to foreign donors and development partners, and also have their limitations.

I need help to scale up anti-FGM work by supporting Usalama's Health Programme. Our main challenge is finding funds for effective implementation of our strategic health objectives and activities.

I also want to establish inter-country exchange programmes, especially with those nations that are already making positive progress in the fight against FGM. For Instance,

I want to see Usalama youth, both men and women interact one-to-one with their counterparts elsewhere, sharing like-minded visions and ideas, and documenting best practices to change the world.

Currently however we don't even have resources to pay the annual renewal fee for our website domain.

We do appreciate that change is a gradual process but with FGM, we can't wait for that gradual change. FGM must stop, yesterday!

....

MEN CAMPAIGNERS

Increasingly, and fortunately, men are becoming more involved in campaigns to eradicate female genital mutilation. The four male campaigners here have in common a concern for the rights and welfare of children and women. Each is also involved professionally in campaigning.

Evanson Njeru, Gerald Lepariyo and Samuel Leadismo emphasise here the issues as seen through the lens of acute concern for their own sisters. All three, with Tony Mwebia, also stress the importance of the rule of law as they seek to encourage family, friends and colleagues, especially the men, to join their fight against FGM.

Evanson Njeru

I have not disclosed all this before, but as I have a platform let me share it now...

FGM has even caused lasting harm in my own family; but, as I will tell, none of my sisters has practised it on their daughters. They have joined hands to say 'no' to FGM, and are on the frontline campaigning against it.

I am a social worker and teacher, now engaged in community development and Director-Founder of Compassion CBO, a Kenyan NGO set up to help people escape from extreme poverty, and which as part of this combats FGM.

I became aware of FGM at the early age of eight years. I knew about it through my great-grandmother who was still alive, and through my grandmother, who were both great proponents of FGM. My Embu community have practiced it as a rite of passage for centuries. In my early years – the early 1980s – it was so strong that no girl could escape the cut. My own parents did not say anything about it and even today have remained dumb, since we lived together with my great-grandmother and my grandma.

When playing with other boys we used to ask each other about it and every one said when we grow up none of us will marry a *Kirigu*, which is the name for an 'uncut' woman. The lives of such women were made very difficult. Our great-grandmother used to say in my family no one will marry a Kirigu and no one will keep a Kirigu. This was a curse she was pronouncing.

This was our world and perception at a young age, because we believed that everything you are told to do by elders is true and good. I did not know which part of the body is circumcised and at that age all I knew was there is boy and girls. It was not clear what makes one to be a girl and another a boy.

My sisters were all at high risk, being the first-born and, below me in the middle, the other two sisters following each other. So I was waiting to see what would happen to them because my great-grandparent died in 1985 when I was barely eleven years old and the curse of a dead person is even more severe than the one for the living. Everybody in the village believed in it.

The ugly part came when FGM touched my own sisters and cousins. My mother, a Christian, was put under heavy pressure and in the end my sisters were snatched from our homestead and taken to an unknown place about seven miles away. When we woke up in the morning I had no sisters.

It was not until 10:00 am the following day that we heard my younger sister was lying on the riverbed because she was still bleeding profusely. She was groaning in pain and my mother was told to go and bring her home. As a young boy aged 15 I ran with others down the steep hill and on the way we met my mother and other women carrying my sister wrapped in *leso* (a piece of cloth).

We were told by my grandparents that the girls had gone under the cut and were now mature. A while later on my sister ran away from school because the teacher refused to teach an adult. We didn't know where she was and we feared she might have killed herself. She returned penniless after six months, but then, still aged just 14, she became pregnant and had a baby girl.

My sister was forced to have FGM, escaping death by a whisker, bleeding profusely and left for worse, but all this helped her to say no to traditional beliefs about the generation curse, and no to FGM for her daughter. Her campaign in the village is 'No to FGM'.

The tradition of female genital mutilation is deeply embedded in my community, not far from Nairobi in Kenya. In Kenya many communities practise FGM. These include the Embu community to which I belong, and my neighbour communities Meru Mbere, Tharaka, Kikuyu and Kamba. These communities are immediate neighbours of Embu. Other distant communities include the Maasai, Samburu, Kisii, Kuria, Nandi and the Coastal tribes, among them the Mijikenda.

Community leaders should be involved in this campaign. Alternative Rites of Passage (ARPs) to FGM should be introduced, like cutting a red ribbon as a symbol of achieving adulthood. Education is very important, as is fighting poverty through income generating activities.

The government should banish the paying of dowries, because many communities practise it so that their daughter can see someone from a different clan to get married in exchange for goods. When I got married I did not pay a dowry because it is a tool used to encourage FGM. This did not go well for me because clan members expected the dowry. Everybody blessed with a daughter anticipates future wealth in the form of dowry.

The laws that criminalise FGM should be implemented and must be followed to the letter. FGM in many communities has gone underground and is currently often unreported.

For example, in our communities in the late 1980s FGM was common and was not criminalised. It was done, not openly like in the '60s and '70s, but it continued. Despite the fear that the government was against FGM, there were then no set policies to fight it. From the later 1990s onwards, due to that fear, the incidence of FGM has begun to decrease.

Then the worst happened, when a sect called Mungiki emerged which influenced the Embu Meru, Tharaka, Mbere and Kikuyu communities. This tobacco snuffing sect subscribed strongly to the cultural beliefs and traditions of the ancestors, including the conduct of worship facing Mount Kenya. In a big way FGM came back again after many youths joined the sect. Members of the 'Mungiki' sect – with an estimated three million followers including many young people – have continuously mutilated their girls.

The financial and other benefits from dowry are why communities cannot be trusted to fight FGM without involving mainstream society. Some communities practise 98 per cent but everything is silent like in the Somali communities. No one talks about it here but people continue to practise it even here near the government offices. Since they are Muslim the media says it's OK, and when the media is silent the government seems silent. But the same knife is used by everyone.

So yes, it is not easy to speak out against FGM because they see you as a traitor. It's like trying to fight drug trafficking. It will hit back. You will be treated as an outcast by some community clan elders, or summoned by elders and fined. You can be bitten or killed by those who benefit from it.

As for the politicians, if you advocate against FGM you are against your community and you will not get votes. You will lose your seat.

Nonetheless, we must come up with laws that stick and make FGM a crime. Anybody caught should be prosecuted and jailed. Others can help by supporting the lobby groups that fight the FGM.

Making FGM history requires personal, community, religious, non-governmental and governmental initiatives. I feel a day can't pass without saying 'No to FGM'.

***

Gerald Lepariyo

I learned about female genital mutilation more than 20 years ago. In 1990 my father told his three daughters (my sisters) that they were about to undergo FGM. This usually happens in December at the end of the year.

Two of my sisters agreed to undergo FGM and one resisted. I remember vividly that my father and other relatives were getting ready to circumcise their girls and a big ceremony was being prepared – only for them to be deeply shocked when they discovered that one of my sisters had escaped during the night, to avoid FGM.

The sister who resisted was chased away from our community, rejected, cursed and denied school. She decided to seek asylum from another neighbouring community called Samburu where she met a woman missionary of the African Inland Church (AIC) who helped her to get into school, and the church managed to pay her school fees.

My sister's refusal was a terrifying time because she was the *only* one in the community who resisted FGM.

This was a real shock to everyone because it had never happened in the history of the community, Ilchamus, from which I come: The Ilchamus (Njemps) are the second smallest community (around 50,000 people) in Kenya, identified as a world minority group. They live around the shores of Lake Baringo. They regard themselves as one of the indigenous communities pushed to the area by Maasai clan wars.

Unfortunately *all* the other girls, who without exception underwent FGM, dropped out of school because of early marriages or as a result of early pregnancies.

The one girl who resisted FGM is the only one who finished secondary school.

Now some of my family members oppose FGM. I myself have a family with one daughter who has said no to FGM. What inspires me most is the photo on my Twitter account, which shows two children, a boy and a girl. These are the twin children of my sister who resisted FGM.

I have undertaken various campaigns despite resistance to stop FGM. I have use media, both electronic and print, and I've carried out sensitisation campaigns, including public barazas (baraza is a Swahili word meaning a deliberative meeting of wise people). I have tried to work with opinion leaders in the community, engaging stakeholders both State and non-State actors to help promote anti-FGM campaigns.

I'm working hard to get support from well-wishers so that I can strengthen our local organisation, the Ilchamus Community Development Trust (ICDT), making it more robust and active in reaching out to families and communities, sensitizing them to the dangers of FGM. We also engage local administration facilities, schools and public barazas as a key focus areas. When used widely with adequate resources these opportunities can really help in terms of creating a greater awareness of the dangers of FGM. Media therefore plays a key role in our sensitisation campaigns.

We must, all together, mobilise resources to help deliver civic education, saving girls by providing them with proper schooling, recruiting more girls to be Ambassadors to say *No to FGM*.

My FGM campaign is a calling from God. It's challenging work because there is a lot of resistance from communities. There is still a fear of victimisation if you speak out.

As you are aware, developing countries still experience profound difficulties in facing up to FGM, especially with Pastoralist and minority communities, because FGM is culturally mandatory for any woman who wants to get married; she must be 'pure'. Remember, marriage among Pastoralists is valued because on marriage women are exchanged for cows as the price of the dowry.

Eradicating FGM will require massive campaigns and funding to be effective. FGM is entrenched at the grassroots in many communities where bride price is very important because of limited resources, and there's a lot of support for the practice. The communities still practising FGM are mostly Pastoralists, who believe men cannot marry a woman who has *not* undergone FGM. These communities are: Ilchamus, Pokots, Samburu, Turkana and Maasai, Rendile and Borana among others.

And so FGM is still rampant in many regions because of male chauvinism, but mainstream society can be active in containing it if serious sensitisation campaigns are undertaken. Educating communities on the dangers of FGM should be the driver for change.

FGM is like Ebola. It can be fatal, and the way global leaders reacted to Ebola absolutely must also be the way to eradicate FGM.

The three fundamental principles of my media campaign work are #EndFGM, #SaveOurGirls, and #SayNoToFGM.

FGM is dangerous. It kills, it's a violation of human rights. It undermines humanity and devalues life. We must end it. Let us support each other and I am sure we will #EndFGM.

***

Samuel Leadismo

All my sisters except one have been through female genital mutilation. My youngest sister who lives with me is not cut. She's in high school. I'm fighting for her right not to be cut.

What I've seen for myself since I was five years old has challenged me to fight this vice. I want to help educate girls and women so they know they are unique, as they were made. I won't go against what God has created. I now have my own family. My wife was circumcised and I've promised not to make my daughter undergo FGM.

With support from Sayydah Garrett, I co-founded the Pastoralist Child Foundation where we educate girls and the community about FGM and child marriage, and we sponsor girls' education. We educate girls about the dangers of the cut, encourage them to stay in school, work hard and pass their examinations to achieve their goals in life.

FGM is generally perceived as barbaric, traumatic and dangerous; but as yet it remains culturally accepted in Samburu County as an important rite of passage despite the harmful side effects. Depending on the precise community, the procedure involves cutting, incision or excision of any part of the female genital organs for cultural, ritual or social purposes.

The Samburu community believes that FGM brings girls to maturity, and afterwards they are forcibly married off and initiated into motherhood. Girls as young as ten years are booked for 'the cut', sometimes with the blessing of their own parents. I saw this happening when I was as young as five years old. In our village, Lorubae, I'd estimate that 98 per cent of our women and girls are cut.

FGM is the main cause of domestic violence among communities who practice it, because when the woman remembers the pain caused by the scar when giving birth, she may decide to sterilise herself without her husband's consent.

FGM shatters girls' dreams of becoming potential leaders in various professional fields.

I don't blame my community because they don't know the real negative impacts of FGM, but we are now trying to educate them. Men who encourage the practice are oblivious to the adverse effects it has on the girls, but I'm a man too, and I am against FGM.

Most of the community here in Samburu is against us campaigners. Sometimes I feel as though I'm not from this community because I'm educating them. They accuse me of wanting to change our culture. But I only want to change the vices in our culture. I will fight for girls' rights and I won't tire of fighting for them.

Circumcision for both boys and girls is one of the most important rituals amongst the Samburu. For boys, circumcision marks the initiation into Moran (warrior) life. For girls, it signifies becoming a woman. Any female in this community who is not circumcised is looked down upon and considered a child, whatever her age. If she gives birth out of wedlock the baby will be killed because the community believes it does not belong to them.

We're also threatened by being cursed by the elders. I don't believe in the curses of the elders. These men are old and known while the majority are younger.

The elders' aim is to ensure that all girls are circumcised before they get married. They give out pocket money to encourage identifying those who have not been cut and those who are therefore suitable for a Samburu Moran to marry. I'd say 90 per cent of Samburu elders and women have difficulty speaking about FGM. Many in my community fear the curses of the elders.

Educating more children in our Samburu community can stop this vice. Pastoralist Child Foundation usually sponsors education for girls from communities that respect our work to eradicate FGM. The girls we sponsor can be the role models of the community.

Barazas (public demonstrations to raise awareness) and big meetings can also help educate our community about FGM. Most Samburu people don't watch the news on TV or have access to any other social media. We live in manyattas (huts) that don't have electricity. There is therefore very limited knowledge of the outside world.

Even now, the practice of FGM sometimes takes place under the supervision of local administration officers such as chiefs, assistant chiefs and district officers. Stern action must be taken against leaders who go contrary to the laws of Kenya and must serve as examples to others. Section 14 of the Children's Act of 2001, clearly states that 'No person shall subject a child to female circumcision, early marriage or other cultural rites, customs or traditional practices that are likely to negatively affect the child's life, health, social welfare, dignity or physical or psychological development.'

The Prohibition of FGM Act of 2011 likewise disallows the 'female cut'. It states that anyone found practicing female circumcision and convicted shall be sent to jail for seven years or fined Kenyan Shillings 500,000 or both. A person who causes death in the process of carrying out female circumcision will be liable to imprisonment for a term of between three to four years or fine of between KSh100,000 and KSh500,000 [£700–3,500 / €980–5,000 / $1,100–5,300].

Nonetheless, FGM continues. Although the majority of people in my community are aware of the dangers and risks associated with female circumcision and forced marriage, they do not as yet link these risks also with the loss of autonomy which girls then experience.

I sometimes feel as though FGM and child marriage are not yet considered a violation of human rights.

So what can we, the Pastoralist Child Foundation (PCF), do to tackle this situation?

We try to educate the Pastoralist communities, we seek to empower Pastoralist women in rural areas, we make a long-term commitment for our girls, we provide boarding school places for our girls and we work with and respect Pastoralist social systems and beliefs, concentrating on the Samburu and Maasai communities.

The Samburu and Maasai communities are two areas with some of the lowest school enrolment levels and highest poverty rates in the country. The education of girls and women is therefore, as in many other socio-economically parallel places, the single most effective way to alleviate poverty.

We provide stability and support for these children. We ensure the girls have sanitary napkins so they can continue school when they start to menstruate, we help to tackle wider problems like access to nutritious meals and clean water, and we offer a place to live and study safe from the prospect of early marriage.

By focussing on the Pastoralist communities' way of life, PCF can address the cultural belief systems, unique to these communities, which prevent girls from being educated. We incorporate the Pastoralist cultural perspective and local concerns into our strategies, thus gaining greater acceptance of our mission among men as well as women.

The Samburu, Pokot, Rendile, and Maasai tribes and many others are still practicing FGM. The practice won't stop immediately. Its eradication requires support from the government, communities and organisations.

***

Tony Mwebia

It was fate that made me aware of female genital mutilation. I was volunteering with an organisation called the HIAS Refugee Trust of Kenya. Then an opportunity arose and they required a project assistant for a pilot project by the United Nations Commissioner for Human Rights (UNHCR), which was meant to educate urban refugees on FGM through community dialogues and sensitisation. Though as a small boy I was aware that FGM was practised in my community, I had never known what it entailed or how it was done.

Being a project assistant, I was required to know all the relevant facts about FGM. This made me do a lot of reading within a very short period of time. By the time I got to the field I thought I had known everything but I was shocked to hear people sharing first-hand information about their experience with FGM. I remember one memorable story of a man narrating how he lost his dear wife during delivery due to complications as a result of FGM. This was the turning point in my life and I vowed to fight FGM by all means possible.

It was not until I was working in Kuria, after I left the HIAS Refugee Trust of Kenya, that I experienced the reality of FGM being performed. In December 2014 to be precise, it was the FGM season among the Kuria community in Kenya. Women sang and danced openly on the road as they escorted their girls to undergo the cut. Young men armed with machetes and spears provided 'security' from the authorities. The police officers were simply overwhelmed by the crowds.

Though for security reasons I could not risk going near, I watched from afar. Many girls underwent the cut and afterwards they walked freely in the market places dressed traditionally to showcase that they had undergone the cut.

My experience from Kuria is that FGM is a communal thing and all the community members are involved in the ceremony especially the dancing procession.

Currently I work with the Child Welfare Society of Kenya as a social worker in Kuria,

Migori County in Kenya. My organisation focuses on tackling different problems and challenges affecting children in Kenya, with FGM being one of them. As a social worker I carry out sensitisation on FGM in chiefs' barazas and other community forums, with the aim of making community members understand the need to abandon this outdated practice.

My own online activism includes #MenENDFGM, which aims at calling upon men from all spheres of life to join in the fight against #FGM. I call urge all men to join in the fight against FGM since it affects our sisters, aunts, friends, cousins, wives and wives to be.

I can't stress enough that not involving men in the fight against FGM is like a doctor treating the symptoms of an illness and ignoring the disease itself.

The only sure way to eradicate FGM in communities is through dialogue and sensitisation aimed at changing people's perceptions and attitudes. From experience, this works in all communities as long as the dialogues are well structured and moderated. The dialogues should be coupled by other projects aimed at improving people's quality of life through education and economic empowerment.

The community here does not really make it difficult for people to speak out. They turn out in large numbers, but once you have spoken, most people rubbish your teachings on their way home. This makes it very difficult since you can be fooled into thinking that everyone is ready for change.

FGM is gradually becoming less common in the Kuria community, but it remains a major challenge. The change has been brought about by constant sensitisation being carried out by NGOs and government agencies. Increased access to education through sponsorship programmes and bursaries has helped in enlightening both boys and girls from this community.

The most appropriate immediate response to FGM for anyone trying to stop harm to a child is to report it to the Sub-county Children's Officers. In most cases this will work; the response is normally good. I will not completely rule out reporting your concerns to chiefs, but this comes with many challenges because some chiefs are deemed to be FGM sympathisers.

This is a national and international problem for the whole world at large and it should not be politicised. It's a problem for all of us. Those who practise FGM are not location-specific. They move around from one region to another through migration. People carry their cultural practises with them as they migrate.

FGM has major economic impacts on society. We all know women are the backbone of our economy. The health complications of FGM drain family resources, as women are bound to require regular treatments in hospitals. Procedures like fistula correction surgery are very expensive. When we expose women to the physical harm and psychological effects of FGM, their productivity is bound to be diminished, at a cost to us all.

THE LAWYER

Christine Nanjala-Ndenga

I am a lawyer with a background in legal aid cases. I now head the prosecution unit on FGM in the Office of the Director of Public Prosecutions in Kenya.

I come from the Luhya tribe in the western part of Kenya and we do not practice FGM. As such I have not experienced it neither have I witnessed it. My secondary school education was however at Moi Girls Isinya High School in Kajiado, in the Rift Valley, where I began hearing stories about FGM from my fellow students. In the 1990s this was something discussed in hushed tones and all that was said was that they cut some of the private parts. I did not give much of a thought to it then.

In Kenya, save for three communities, all the rest have a history of practising FGM. The differences arise from the type of cutting, which varies from one community to another, but it had not happened to my own family members.

Moving forward, things have changed, and I am very involved in legal activities aimed at stopping FGM. I must confess this was not a field I thought I would work in when I joined the Office of the Director of Public Prosecutions. I thank God for giving me this commission and the Director of Public Prosecution for allowing me to take the task forward.

The ODPP Unit is engaged in community and public education programmes as well as prosecuting cases on FGM under the *Prohibition of FGM Act 2011*. So far the team has been quite instrumental, having visited 16 counties that have a high prevalence of FGM based on the *2008–09 Kenya Demographic and Health Survey*, which was supported by the United Nations, the World Bank and some other agencies.

The ODPP FGM Unit recently developed a report, intended for dissemination from March 2015, and leading to a National Stakeholder Forum for state and non-state actors on FGM in Kenya.

The Unit is also undertaking prosecution of FGM cases in Kenya. These are interesting offences to prosecute and very personal as well as emotional.

I must confess that the journey of the past year has been more of a learning experience above all else for the team.

During the time I have been actively involved in this campaign FGM has been on my mind continuously. It has not affected me at first hand, but I have traversed the country and seen the impact of FGM on the women and girls. I have witnessed deaths and I am currently prosecuting cases related to this.

I am focussing on how Kenya can move towards abandonment of the practice.

My thoughts are concerned with creating synergies among all actors and analysing strategies that can achieve abandonment of FGM. I guess I have reached a point where I want to see people move. I want to see results ... I would really love to see results.

Kenya has employed a multifaceted approach in tackling issues of FGM. This has included public education on the effects and impacts of FGM, creating public awareness on the legislation and recently prosecution under the law. Kenya is currently re-defining the message for the campaigns, towards behaviour and attitude change in the societies that practice FGM.

Prosecution is also one of the ways that the issues of FGM can be tackled.

Education to create awareness of issues of FGM, especially for the young girls, is also crucial.

Unfortunately the efforts in Kenya on issues like FGM are compartmentalised. There is as yet no synergy in the service delivery. That said we believe that counselling, education (specifically sex and FGM education), reproductive health services and victim and witness support are salient.

We need a referral system for victims and those at risk that actually works.

One serious worry is the trends towards medicalisation of FGM, which is becoming entrenched among some communities. It is important that we rope the medical practitioners into the campaigns against FGM.

I want to believe the practice of FGM in Kenya is on the decline. My fear however is that this decline may just be a facade as the practice in other areas has gone underground. The issue of cross border practice is also rife.

Without proper statistics on the emerging trends it is difficult to establish the real prevalence of FGM; and accompanying FGM are other harmful practices such as early marriage, denial of the right to education and reproductive rights, and honour killings (though not normally referred to as that).

We need to have a message that moves towards behaviour change and changes in social attitudes. With continued engagement some communities have now begun speaking out. However in my own assessment there are other locations in Kenya where discussion of FGM remains a taboo.

All of society should have a say in issues of FGM. The communities inter-marry and this practice affects us all in one-way or another. Everyone needs to recognise that FGM is not a class issue.

Just like any other element in society the practise of FGM is struggling to remain relevant and as a result it keeps on changing every single day.

Pulling together government agencies and civil society can produce a louder voice that cannot be ignored by decision makers. Most urgent on my agenda for this year (2015) is to bring all actors together to foster collaboration.

The media and others can help us here. I want to see every single success story highlighted to give hope to those in this field. Best practices must be documented, failures openly acknowledged, and all the lessons learnt from what we do must be shared and inculcated into new interventions.

As long as I am in this field, I will keep trying, hoping the little we are doing is making a life better.

. . . .

The work of these Kenyan campaigners continues. You can read more news about their work via the Female Mutilation Worldwide website. We will also discover as we read on here that some of the Kenyan activists who have already shared their experiences are supported by people from other parts of the world.

Sayydah Garrett and Teri Gabrielsen, for instance, are North Americans who co-founded a campaign to eradicate female genital mutilation, after chance encounters with elders of traditionally practising communities whilst on quite separate safaris in Kenya. Sayydah joined forces with Samuel Leadismo (above) and Teri now collaborates with another local leader, James Ole Kamete. Likewise, Cath Holland is a British midwife who spends much of her time in Kenya. She has a close association with Domtila Chesang (also above) and is a founder of the charity, Beyond FGM.

Cath, Sayydah and Teri all support programmes to introduce Alternative Rites of Passage (ARPs) as a harmless and positive way to celebrate girls achieving adult status; and all are adamant that more support and funding must be made available for those who work 'on the ground' with communities, if FGM is finally to be eradicated. The most effective ways to eradicate FGM vary significantly, however, between different locations. As we shall see in the next chapter, which focuses on a global region, because of history and tradition FGM is in some places perceived by those who do it to be a formal religious obligation.

CHAPTER 4:

Sub-Saharan and Southern Africa

The received wisdom has been that female genital mutilation occurs mainly in the Sub-Saharan belt of Africa, but more recently we have realised that FGM has also occurred for many centuries elsewhere, including other regions of Africa and, as we shall see (Chapter 5), in the Middle East and some parts of Asia. Customs can move with people, sometimes over vast distances. Rationales or beliefs, and how things are done, may change, but the fundamentals of the act itself often do not. Pervasive, unquestioning traditional modes of behaviour and understandings present major challenges when it comes to eradicating FGM.

In this chapter our quest to learn more about FGM takes us West to East across central Africa, and then in a southerly direction until we reach Malawi.

SIERRA LEONE

F.A. Cole and Hawa Sesay are survivors of FGM, both born in Sierra Leone, where over 90 per cent of women are subject to the practice. Mr A is also Sierra Leonean by birth. F.A. (Francess) Cole, a successful speaker and author, now lives in the United States (Chapter 7); and Hawa Sesay, also a campaigner, lives in the UK (Chapter 9), as does Mr A, who here speaks very candidly about his personal experience of the impacts on intimacy when a partner has been subject to female genital mutilation.

***

F.A. Cole

I was eleven years old when my father and stepmother decided my older sister and I should go through FGM, a horrific rite of passage into womanhood. It happened in August 1984 at the Bondo Bush located off Savage Street in the capital city of Freetown in Sierra Leone, West Africa. I don't know by whom it was performed because I was blindfolded.

This excerpt from my autobiography *Distant Sunrise – The Strength in her Pain to Forgive* explains what happened:

"Upon arriving at the place where we would be made into women, we were greeted with hails of happy chants and traditional songs by about a dozen women. [My sister] Malaika and I greeted them in our local dialect (Krio) and we were led into the hut to be striped of our clothes. The ""bondo bush" where so many vicious acts have occurred, had a massive tree in the center of the compound and a small hut made of zinc with thatched roof at the far right. The hut had no rooms just an open space with two twin-size mattresses; one casually thrown on the muddy floor. Forget about modern amenities such as a bathroom and toilet. If we felt like going we did it in the paint can and someone was responsible for emptying and cleaning it, what a job. Well, we did it for nine days, and when it was time for us to take a shower, we had water drawn for us in a bucket and we stood in one corner of the compound to shower. This I did not mind doing, as I was only eleven years old. Back to that dreadful night in question. After we were stripped completely, they led us to sit on a mat underneath the tree while they prepared the "ritual bed." Upon completion, Malaika, because she was the older was called on first and I was given strict warnings not to turn around.

Sitting on the ground, head slightly bent forward, I tried to make sense of what was happening to my dear angel amid the shouting and howling. After what seemed like centuries, Malaika joined me under the tree, tears rolling down her cheeks. Like a sheep being led to the slaughter house, I was led to the "ritual bed." Before anything could be done to me, I was blind folded and my hands tied behind my back. With the help of an unknown woman, I was forced to lie on the "bed" face up; and from that moment the worse nightmare of my life began. As I lay helplessly, my legs were widely spread apart and pinned down by two women while another sat on top of me. A woman ten times my size sat on top of my chest. This was the least of my pains. After she sat on her human bench made of the limp body of an eleven year-old girl, she was handed the weapon of death. To this day I can't tell if they used the same razor blade used on Malaika, but one thing I know is that it was not sterilized nor was I given any form of anaesthesia. As she held my little clitoris between her fingers and the blade in the other hand, I started to wiggle under her. Seeing I would be trouble if I was not securely pinned down, others joined in to restrain me..."

"As she began to cut, I screamed and fought with all my might, and in the process of all this an opportunity presented itself and I jumped at it. Fully utilizing the only weapon I had, I pulled my head forward with the little strength I had left in me and mercilessly bit into her buttock as she herself was naked. Thereafter, I was gagged to stop the screams. I must have lost more than a pint of blood. After the cutting, the women who held me down pulled me to my feet but because I had lost so much blood I felt catatonic and could barely walk. As I was being led to sit on the mat underneath the tree, I looked down and to my dismay, realised I was covered in blood from my hips downward. This was, and still is one of the most disturbing things I have ever seen. It felt like I was walking on broken glass and hot coals and those witches refused to carry me. So, tightly gripping their arms, I tipped toed to the tree and gently sat on the mat with my legs widely spread apart. To slowly stop the bleeding, we had a string of rope tied around our waist and a piece of cloth (in place of a menstrual pad) placed between our legs (like a loin cloth.) Malaika and I sat in silence and in excruciating pain whilst they jubilated. Before going any further, let me explain that each time blood is shed it is sign of a covenant. To what or whom we were offered as a sacrifice I do not know, but know that I was in bondage for a very long time. A part of me was cut off and blood was shed and since this is their "tradition" and prayers were made to some gods before they started the process, that part of me was offered to something and it held onto it. I take a moment to thank God for delivering me from spiritual bondage and for giving me the opportunity to share my story. It is a taboo to disclose this information to "non-members" (but thank God, I am not a member and can therefore share my story with nothing to fear.) For *"if God be for you who can be against you"* And according to 1John 4:4 *"ye are of God little children, for greater is He that is in you than he that is in the world."* (KJV) To this day, I have no idea what was done with my clitoris. Was it buried? Given to their gods? Thrown in the nearby stream? Or was it (as most people in my country believe) cooked in cassava or potato leaves with fish and palm oil and given us to eat? I have absolutely no idea. However, I hope it was not the latter."

I learned later, from my sister after publishing *Distant Sunrise*, that Papa may have regretted his decision because the grandmother of our cook's daughter wanted to take the girl (her granddaughter) for FGM but Papa refused to have her go through it. My mum who is Creole didn't go through this nonsense so there really is nothing to discuss with her.

FGM is still being practiced in Sierra Leone, but mostly in the provinces. Based on responses to my questions I learned FGM is still practiced in Freetown but it is not as popular as it once was – like twenty years ago. The reason for this decline is due to education on the impacts of FGM.

These communities brainwash victims into believing that if they ever share the 'secret' with anyone, they'll die. The reason for secrecy is that FGM is not viewed as a violation, rather it is believed to be a secret society and what's done in the Bondo Bush should be kept secret.

It is important to understand two things.

Firstly, FGM is a money-making industry because the women who do the 'cutting' are paid cash and they also receive gifts such as expensive jewellery, alcohol, expensive African cloths, etc.

Secondly, FGM is a demonic practice. It serves no purpose in the lives of its victims. I later learned that our clitorises are chopped off in order to 'control' our sexual urges and cause us to be 'faithful' to one man – our husband. Hmmm ... can anyone control another's sexual urges?

My message to decision makers in Sierra Leone is this:

'God created girls with a clitoris for a specific reason and nowhere in His Word does He say we should have it amputated. Forcefully subjecting young girls and teenagers to this horrific practice is a gross violation of our human rights and no amount of therapy can reverse the traumas brought on by this practice.

'Think about the lifelong implications: painful menstrual periods; painful sexual intercourse; maternal mortality; unnecessary tearing during child birth, etc ... is this something you would want to have your daughters suffer for the rest of their lives?

'How would you feel if one of your basic human rights were violated? God gave each individual the will to choose but in our case, we were not given the opportunity to say yes or no. It is time you stand up for the rights of children and girls and let them live a life of peace and love. The pains, frustration, bitterness, anger and low self-esteem brought on by FGM can never be erased. That type of human cruelty is very difficult to forgive because the scars (physical and psychological) stay with those who survive.

'There should be stricter laws to prosecute and punish anyone (parents, grandparents, cutters, etc) found guilty of subjecting girls to this barbaric practice.

'Make FGM and its impacts part of the curriculum in primary and secondary schools and train community leaders on that as well. Help the people understand that girls can still go through a harmless rite of passage and be trained on the roles of women in their society... this can be done away from the "bondo bushes" and, instead, in classroom settings.

'And please create and encourage support groups within communities for survivors and their families...'

I now live in the USA. I am involved in activities to bring awareness about, and to stop, FGM. I am not part of any grass roots groups but I do get invited to share my story of surviving FGM and other forms of sexual violence. I then use these opportunities to point people to organisations and grass roots groups and encourage them to get involved.

I launched my foundation *F.A. Cole* and a magazine, *LifeAfter FGM*, in March 2015. The magazine will be based solely on interviewing survivors of FGM. God gave me this divine idea in December 2014, on my way to church. A lot of us are working tirelessly to stop FGM but no one is actually talking to or with survivors of FGM on what life is like after FGM. I would love to work with campaigners like Alimatu Dimonekene, Hilary Burrage, The Girl Generation, GirlChildNetwork Sierra Leone, Ifrah Ahmad and others.

I want to use LifeAfter FGM as a platform for survivors of FGM and other forms of sexual violence to share their stories of survival and encourage others to do the same. I want to explain to girls that they should not live in fear of being ostracised by their family or communities for speaking out against FGM.

Unfortunately, I am not aware of any services to support survivors. For support we survivors can rely on each other. We do not need sympathy, just love and support in ending FGM.

We need to talk about it. Sharing brings healing, one speech at a time. We must help survivors understand that there's nothing to be ashamed of or feel guilty about. What happened to them is not because they did something wrong but due to the ignorance of their people.

I have T-shirts made that read 'I survived Female Genital Mutilation' and I wear them to events where I know I'll run into people who've never heard of FGM. I use that opportunity to share my story and encourage them to join in the fight to end FGM any way they can.

You may choose not to go that route but there are other ways you can support us in this fight. Search for organisations and grass roots groups working to end FGM in your area and volunteer your time or money.

***

Hawa Sesay

I underwent female genital mutilation – which local people call 'Sunna' – at the age of 13, in my home village in Sierra Leone. I was blindfolded, as if it was an execution, because that is the tradition to avoid the cutter being identified, but I know in fact that the practitioner was my aunt.

I was also gagged, to stop crying out, as it is thought weak for a girl to cry or shout. If you make a noise you are not a strong woman, and then there are complaints to your family. The reality however is that the pain is so intense you think you are dying.

Most girls are cut around the harvest time, which in Sierra Leone is, in Western schedules, the Christmas, or sometimes the Easter, holidays.

If a family plans to migrate, or send children, to another country, FGM is usually done before they leave Sierra Leone, which is easier than sending girls back 'home'.

FGM is required by the secret Bondo or Sande Societies, which operate respectively in the North and South of Sierra Leone. The tradition goes back many centuries and is very difficult to challenge. People are afraid of the secret societies and what they can do to you.

Politicians who question FGM are likely to find they are not re-elected because the secret societies ensure they don't get votes. This is also why imprisonment for FGM is infrequent, even though Sierra Leone's 2007 child rights legislation is clear that any practice which 'dehumanises or is injurious to the physical or mental welfare of a child' is strictly illegal.

The one fact everyone knows about me is my background, that I will never make a secret of female genital mutilation. The culture of silence and denial around child abuse must end. I know from my own experience how difficult it is for victims to speak up, so when they do, it is vital that we listen, believe, and treat them with respect.

After I came to the UK, I set up the Hawa Trust Ltd as a community interest company. It is a grassroots local organisation working in Hackney, London, among African and other ethnic minority communities, with a specific focus on the Sierra Leonean community. The Trust works to support communities in tackling FGM, to engage with them to change attitudes, to provide information for young women and girls, and to provide referrals to other organisations and statutory services.

Amongst the matters I am working on in Hackney are human trafficking and FGM, with AFRUCA (Africans United Against Child Abuse), and the FGM telephone helpline which the National Society for the Prevention of Cruelty to Children (NSPCC) organised.

I also advise the Royal College of Midwives and various government bodies on FGM. There are a lot of issues still to be addressed, for instance, how do we refer women and girls with FGM to hospitals for treatment, when there is a risk that this will become a criminal matter and perhaps someone they know or depend on will be imprisoned?

I've learned that people will forget what you said, and forget what you did; but they will never forget how you made them feel. I will not forget the day I was cut.

I didn't talk about FGM and the harm it has done me when I first came to the UK, but now I work hard to stop it. My own daughter only asked what I know about FGM when she was already a teenager, and she was deeply shocked by what I had to tell her.

***

Mr A

I was born in Sierra Leone where I spent my formative years, before moving to the UK in 1993. FGM is prevalent in Sierra Leone, with the World Health Organisation (WHO) estimating that 88 per cent of women may have undergone the practice. It is amongst the very few countries where FGM explicitly still has not been completely banned.

I became aware of FGM at age 13 – during cultural studies at history lesson in Year 9. Sierra Leone has 17 ethnic groups and all with the exception of one group, the Creoles, practice FGM. I am a Creole hence the delay in my consciousness of a practice I was not acquainted with.

It was not until I moved over to the UK, first in 1999 and then again in 2005, that I had a direct, personal experience of women surviving with FGM. I later came to know that both my partners would have undergone what is classified as a Type 2 procedure.

I've a somewhat vague recollection about my first experience. My partner always complained of pain and dryness during sexual intercourse, but she was very reluctant to discuss the effect FGM was having on her wellbeing, and she was seemingly defensive of the practice.

My second experience over five years was rather different. It was a much more intimate relationship with a partner who opposes FGM. She had not had any previous intimate relationship, so I was able to experience how she became very distressed during intercourse right from the onset. Unlike my first relationship there was no experience of dryness, but my second partner complained of chronic and enduring pain during intercourse. She also experienced relentless subnormal pain during her menstrual cycle.

My second partner was much more open about her experience. She told me that her mother, herself not a victim, married into an ethnic group that practiced FGM. Her father was also, despite his ethnicity, opposed to the practice and it was her aunty, her father's sister, who took her and her little sister without her parents' consent to be circumcised when they went to spend time with her. This later caused a family feud between my partner's parents and the aunt.

From my point of view as a man, sex enhances bonding and improves emotional connection between partners. The absence of the pleasure of sex does affect such experiences. The emotional baggage and barriers (the unpleasant sexual experience) that accompany FGM do create challenges in relationships

The decision makers in my country of origin are very weak. FGM is an integral cultural practice widely accepted by the general population in Sierra Leone. Critical reviews of problems in legislating against the practice make the point that legislation and criminal sanctions in nations where the prevalence of FGM is high maybe unsuccessful, if the majority of the society believe that FGM serves the common good.

The good will is lacking in Sierra Leone as leaders will pay a very heavy price politically should they attempt to legislate fully against FGM.

....

NIGERIA

Nigeria has the highest absolute number of people with FGM of anywhere in the world, because its population is so large. The proportion of women and girls who have undergone FGM is about 30 per cent, so best estimates suggest more than 19 million Nigerians have experienced FGM. Some Nigerian states have previously outlawed FGM explicitly, but it is only this year that the outgoing President, Goodluck Jonathan, decreed that the practice is illegal throughout the country.

Olutosin Oladosu Abedowale is a survivor of female genital mutilation. She was born and works in Nigeria, where she is a writer and activist on women's issues.

Olutosin Oladosu Adebowale

I was born and continue to live in Nigeria. As a child in Ondo State, female genital mutilation was performed for children (not babies) in groups by an elderly woman or man. FGM was referred to as 'ja dodo' in our local dialect and it was quite normal to see young girls aged seven and above showing the wound to their friends. We lived a communal life so we are all related by blood, as distant or close relatives.

What I can remember was that FGM was performed in groups, the herbalist who did it in those days usually used the edge of a very big snail shell to cut the genitals. Girls would then be walking as if there was an object in between their laps.

The herbalists were held in high regards in those days. They were the intermediaries between men and the gods, so there was no disapproval of their actions. It was seen then as a favour to the children and their families, not as business like nowadays.

FGM doesn't bother me personally because I don't know what I would have been without it, so I have accepted my fate. I do however think that FGM reduces sexual pleasure. That is true.

I am now 42 and I have a family of my own. My family and my work as a women's rights activist are what is important to me. I write about women issues and FGM is one of the issues. The social media – Facebook, Twitter, World Pulse and Safe World for Women – all help me to get my message out to a wider audience.

My duty is to write about FGM and expose the secrecy. I've never been involved in any direct activity to end FGM. I am the founder of the Star of Hope Transformation Center in Lagos. We work with abused women and we have a story book library for children, amongst others.

The Nigerian government does not make adequate information about FGM available to citizens. The herbalists have enough misinformation to reign amongst the people. I have had opportunities to travel to different parts of Nigeria. It's the same story everywhere.

To eradicate FGM in the communities in Western Nigeria, it is crucial to educate the herbalists, missionary midwives in churches and nurses who perform this dastardly act in their homes. The custodians of harmful practices currently have better information than the health workers. It's sad.

FGM is no longer acceptable in my town, Owo, because the people are afraid of being arrested by the police, but in other towns in my State (Ondo) in Western Nigeria, FGM is still practised daily.

I have been visiting a town called Oka Akoko in Western Nigeria to investigate an alleged case of FGM. All the men said that a girl had been mutilated but all the women denied it. I need to discover the real facts, because in another village all the women were under a terrible oath not to talk about FGM. In that village FGM is only performed on pregnant women and newly wedded brides.

Mainstream society must be active in stopping FGM. If you leave ending FGM to the custodians of the practice, it will remain forever.

There are also several other traditional harmful practices of which I am aware. These include:

- Witch-mobbing / killing / hunting
- Son-preference
- Widowhood's rites in Eastern Nigeria, where some women are forced to drink the water that was used to bathe the corpse of her husband- just to prove her innocence
- Widow's disinheritance
- In some families in Western Nigeria a woman who newly delivers a baby will eat *lizards* for seven days
- In a village where pregnant women's genitals are cut, they have a peculiar tradition where the language of women is different from the language of men. A son who speaks the language of his mother will be disowned. Both parents are from the same village though, the language of women is like that of a slave
- Incision to cure witchcraft and convulsion is practiced in western Nigeria
- A very horrible practice in some western part of Nigeria is making sure that a woman sleeps with a widower every night in order to separate him from the dead wife. I saw a man who refused this act in 2014, a very young man who claimed to love his dead wife, and he was relocated from his rented apartment; that is the solution. For a man who has no money to relocate, it would be a big problem.

In the traditionally practising communities with which I am familiar it's still difficult to speak out because FGM is linked to God. I want people to share the articles I've written so everyone knows more about FGM in Nigeria. FGM thrives in secrecy.

The Nigerian Government must create a department for FGM and other harmful practices, and do research, to produce findings about how to stop FGM for Nigerians.

My dream for 2015 is to start a documentary called #touchinglives, going to villages to document issues about women and solving these issues. I will need financial support to implement my plan. It's never been done before but I can do it.

....

SOMALIA

Very nearly all women in Somalia have experienced FGM. Legal prohibition remains very weak, even in those parts where it exists at all. Hibo Wardere grew up in Somalia and is a survivor of FGM. Now a mother of four, she lives in the UK (Chapter 9) and has recently been appointed as an End FGM Co-ordinator for the London Borough of Waltham Forest.

Ahmed Hassan was born in Somalia and is Director of Action for Women and Children Concern (AWCC), a not-for-profit organisation which fights violence against women and children in Somalia. He now lives in Minnesota, USA (Chapter 7). Although men in Somalia are not supposed to know about FGM, Ahmed was always aware of this women's issue and is fundamentally opposed to it.

***

Hibo Wardere

Being circumcised was I thought an honour. I was only six years old. Every little girl in our area had been circumcised but I and few others were not. The other girls would tease us about it and also sing as well. I started asking my mum: I wanted it done so that nobody would tease me, or worse not play with me because I had not been cut. So mum was extremely happy that I decided to be circumcised. Little did I know this would cause unimaginable pain? After two days I was to be circumcised.

My mum bought me a new dress to wear afterwards. That morning mum woke me up early in the morning, gave me a bath and breakfast and said 'the ladies are coming', so all the females in my house gathered started singing and I thought I was the centre of attention and enjoyed it. The ladies came. There were about three of them, quite big and fat really. One sat down and told me to sit on her. So I did. Straight away she put both her hands under my armpits and held me tight. One of my aunties held one of my legs very tight and the other leg was held by the other lady.

To cut the story short, they butchered me. I felt I was going to die. In fact I prayed to die.

My whole body was trembling from head to toe. For days I was in great pain. To pass a wee was the worst pain ever.

After ten days I was getting better. For years I suffered flash backs and waking up in the middle of the night sweating and breathing really hard as if It was happening to me there and then. The physical pain that comes from that is quite powerful.

Later you start to think about when you will get married and whether greater pain awaits you. Then you think about when I become a mother. I would be experiencing another pain. All I could think about was, my life is full or is going to be full of pain.

Then I started to feel resentment towards my mother and thinking why, why, why would she let this happen? I thought mums loved their children and that they would never let any harm come to them. I thought she was my protector, apart from God. I still have flash backs now and then.

When I became 15 years old I told my mother I will never ever let any of my daughters go through what I went through. My mum's reaction to that was, 'We will take your daughters to have them circumcised, there's no question about it'. She said, 'I circumcised you so that you wouldn't get off with any boy until you get married, then your husband would be pleased and our honour would be intact, as it has been for generations before you.'

This shouldn't be happening, ever. Medically, forever afterwards you get infections most of the time. Giving birth is dangerous too, because you don't have enough vaginal lips to expand. Instead you will be cut both sideways and downwards – which I can tell you from first-hand experience is the most horrendous pain ever.

Even today where the parent knows there is no 'need' for FGM, they still do it to the innocent little girls.

To these parents the only thing that matters is the family honour.

***

Ahmed Hassan

Fortunately (though I don't know whether it is good word to use in this context), I am male, and as a male person I was not supposed to know about female genital mutilation. In my country we men don't ask when and where it is happening.

As I am writing this now, a girl may be going through FGM somewhere in my homeland or region. We at Action for Women and Children Concern (AWCC) work to stop this in Somalia, and in the Somalian community in the USA.

Traditionally, the event is dominated by women. From its starting point, it is women who organise it. Days before the FGM operation is to be carried out on a certain victim, her family invites relatives and friends to participate in the event or 'service'. Girls undergo FGM in their pre-teens, usually just before their tenth birthday.

There is a small prayer ritual conducted ahead of the FGM operation, usually the evening before the FGM day. The rituals focus on prayers for the girl's common good.

Our culture means that men don't participate in the FGM event. For men it is always taboo to see girls' genitals, but they are aware of what the women may be doing.

In my childhood I can remember seeing girls whose legs were put in shackles ('*Dabar*') to ensure the recovery process, which is strictly observed. The practitioners who perform FGM are nurses, traditional birth attendants (TBAs) or midwives.

The female members of the family, and their neighbours, relatives and friends, all participate and are involved in the event. They participate in the preceding rituals, visit whilst the operation is taking place, and congratulate the FGM victims, paying continued visits during the recovery days after the FGM operation. Some of the visitors give money to the FGM victim to encourage the practice.

I knew of the existence of FGM ever since I was able to recognise things in my childhood. Initially as a child, like other children I was growing up with, I thought it was permissible, but as of the beginning of millennium I was sure it has no room in human rights and has dire consequences for a girl's survival, as well as for the socio-economic conditions of the community.

Men are abetting the continuation of the practice. Women who have not undergone the FGM are likely to be divorced on the first day of their honeymoon. The belief is that if women have not undergone FGM they are not virgin. AWCC explains that FGM victims can still become promiscuous, or not, as they choose.

We are trying to persuade families not to disown women who may have been divorced simply because they have not undergone FGM. Girls without FGM may end up being ostracised, so the consequence of not undergoing FGM is far worse even than the pain of FGM through her entire life. This makes the girls want to undergo FGM.

In the meantime, there is the cultural practice when women/girls fight and insult each other ('*Soo Feedo*'). They ask each other to strip in public to demonstrate they are virgin and have not been involved in sex before marriage - and the interpretation of virginity is very much linked with FGM.

So, if any girl fails to strip in public to present her virginity as evidenced by FGM, it will be shame for her and her entire family. This practice therefore also encourages the FGM.

And in the meantime we also continue to harness knowledge on FGM's socio-economic impact.

FGM has direct impact on our vision in achieving equality in the education sector. You cannot reduce gender disparity in education unless you have a good number of girls in classes, and FGM is a challenge to this. We show our communities the effects of FGM on education and hope that someday all communities will recognise this, as some already have.

We are currently thinking about an innovative approach to reach out to women, because it is they who are the victims and it is disproportionately they who contribute to the perpetuation of FGM.

Our approach is Women To Women (W2W), an idea we will be sharing with our friends and board members in the USA as a concept to be developed. With this approach we will recruit influential women to conduct house calls to sensitise women to get rid of FGM.

It seems we are currently missing role models. Significant institutions like the Somalian government and other political groups are not serious about ending the practice. Politicians and high figures in the limelight in Somalia practice the FGM, but when they speak on the media they say different things to convince donors and Western allies.

Sadly, FGM is not becoming less common. It is practiced just as in years before. This is because advocacy is not going the right approach. For example you will see billboards erected in Mogadishu (Somalia's capital city) and in urban areas, with the message written in English. But people are highly illiterate and they don't speak English anyway.

The question then is, who are such billboards for? Will they deliver the message?

Can it be that NGOs using this approach want to convince the donors, rather than achieving FGM advocacy? These billboards will not end the practice.

Nonetheless, speaking out is not difficult within communities. You can speak out about FGM, but they will present difficult questions, such as who will be taking responsibility for girls divorced on the first night of their honeymoon for not being virgin because they have not undergone FGM?

And who prevents girls from being promiscuous, if they have not undergone FGM?

Our hope is that the planned W2W approach will shine a light on all of these difficult issues.

To practice what they preach, we want the Somali President and the Prime Minister and other high ranking people within the political spectrum, as well as Somali celebrities, to state clearly and demonstrate by example that their children and family members have not undergone and will not undergo FGM.

The media is watching and will cover the stories if these people secretly perform FGM, so by acting as they preach the decision makers can be role models.

The problem is that Somali politicians and political groups rely for election on clan support, so for them to embrace what clans consider taboo may tarnish their image, and they would lose their clan's votes. Nonetheless, we need politicians to ignore clan support and be committed to the documents they signed with the UN and international treaties.

This duplicity by some influential people is derailing our work to stop FGM in Somalia. Other leaders however do make sure we are heard; they promote our work and get us invited to international meetings where we can present our ideas and approaches.

We as an organisation want to be heard internationally and to get support from international countries to continue our advocacy to change in our communities – not only or just FGM, but all sexual and gender-based violence.

....

UGANDA

Ahabwe Mugerwa Michael was born and works in Uganda, where FGM is illegal and found only in a few and mostly isolated communities. He founded the Integrated Community Efforts for Development (ICOD) Action Network. One focus of Ahabwe's work (he is also known as 'Michael') is the ICOD 'Barefoot Grannies' programme, which campaigns to end female genital mutilation in rural areas of Uganda such as Karamoja, a region with around twice the maternal and infant mortality rates for Uganda as a whole. Other core ICOD concerns include obstetric fistula and cross-border trafficking.

Ahabwe Mugerwa Michael

A few years ago I was at a health camp hosted by the organisation I founded, the Integrated Community Efforts for Development (ICOD) Action Network, and I met an FGM victim with obstetric fistula, a condition that devastates the life of women affected by it. This lady shared with me and the rest of our staff her story about FGM and how it had resulted in the fistula. For me this was a turning point; it inspired me to learn more about what FGM victims go through. I think this experience laid a foundation for my current work in eradicating FGM.

Since that meeting I have been very concerned about women and girls in East Africa who live with FGM, and in April 2012 I travelled to Eastern Uganda to talk to people who had been subjected to it. I have also remained in touch with that first woman I met, back in 2012. She is my hero. Her willingness to share her story introduced me to one of the best things that have shaped my activism about women rights and reproductive health.

My first experience of work in the community was as a volunteer, in my home town whilst I was still at school. I had a placement with a big non-governmental organisation developing an HIV/AIDS support programme. This gave me a lot of exposure to such problems, and after I left school I trained and worked as a social worker.

A little later, I decided to take forward my own organisation, the Integrated Community Efforts for Development (ICOD) Action Network, because I wanted to be directly involved in solving the most pressing challenges facing my community, such as

HIV/AIDS and famine and food security.

I am glad to report that since then I've seen ICOD grow from a small volunteer-based group to a national organisation with substantial programmes.

I coordinated and supervised the first health camp and I have coordinated many more since 2008.

We use these health camps to extend health services to people who would not have got such services. We work with medical doctors to treat common illnesses, carry our surgeries and offer dental services. Most people who benefit from our health camps are poor and vulnerable, and can't afford medical costs or the costs of transport to travel to health centres.

I usually organise all the activities of the camp, including for instance the arrival times for visiting doctors to co-ordinate with when we have foreign doctors taking part. I am still in my early thirties and don't have a family of my own because I am not yet married, but I come from a large family of four sisters and three brothers. My family is very important to me and they have all been supportive, helping to welcome and host the foreign interns and volunteers visiting our work in Uganda.

One of our responses to the continuing tragedy of FGM has been to develop the Barefoot Grannies programme. This is an association of eight grassroots organisations of elderly women and mothers in Uganda's Karamoja region. We (ICOD Action Network) are working with these organisations to promote women's reproductive health.

The 219 grannies and mothers who comprise our Barefoot Grannies group are becoming exceptional visionaries who can change their communities through technical support, resource allocation and network building, emphasizing especially FGM and reproductive health issues.

We choose to work with Barefoot Grannies because we believe that strengthening local capacity will ensure sustainability of our work and that of other development partners working to eradicate FGM. Grassroots activism and work in communities where FGM is rampant can also help eradicate the practice. I think working with and supporting small grassroots organisations can help build sustainable local capacity to eradicate the practice.

I honestly believe that the eradication of FGM would also eliminate obstetric fistula. FGM is a major cause of obstetric fistula and urethral damage. In the communities I am familiar with FGM is carried out by cutters with no medical backgrounds and they use one knife on several girls and women. In cases like these, chances are above 90 per cent for victims to develop fistula over time.

I have personally met several women with fistula and seen how severe it can get. I think no person who meets women like these can remain the same. This is the reason we are working on addressing post-FGM effects like fistula.

In addition to ICOD's direct involvement in activities to stop FGM I have strongly come out to advocate for men's direct involvement in reproductive health issues in Uganda. I am encouraging men to take part actively in efforts to end female genital mutilation.

If we are to achieve sustainable results in anti-FGM work, I think men must also be fully engaged in ending it. Instead, it is currently often the case in communities that practice FGM that men actually promote it, arguing that women who have been 'cut' make better wives.

The traditionally held values about sex, gender and FGM make it very hard to publically speak out against FGM in communities I am familiar with. In some communities, it's still unusual to find men advocating for women in matters such as sexual and reproductive rights.

I have myself encountered hostility in some villages, but I've always found ways to put it aside. I hope this will inspire more men to join anti-FGM campaigns.

FGM bothers me so much. What's so frustrating is the fact that the practice is on the rise in remote communities in East Africa despite efforts by civil society organisations and local governments. Girls and women are not informed about their rights, or about the protection provided by the available legislations.

Promoters of FGM have little regard (if any) for girls' and women's lives lost, or for the health complications that victims experience after undergoing FGM. Some local political leaders are afraid to publicly condemn the practice for fear of losing elections; they may even seek to protect offenders.

There is cross-border illegal trafficking of girls between Uganda and Kenya in the areas where FGM is still practised. This has made efforts to end FGM in remote border communities very hard.

There is a real need to create rapid response facilities, both to track and rescue girls before they are forced to undergo FGM and / or forced marriages, and to deliver health and psychological support for victims trafficked across the border.

Early care and treatment of health complications like fistula and paralysis are critical elements in improving quality of life for victims, and such services also help everyone to perceive the grim consequences of FGM.

Traditional beliefs about FGM in remote and highly illiterate regions are some of the reasons for the rise in the practice despite efforts by different partners. I think it will take quite a lot of time to bring everyone in these communities on board in working to end FGM.

It's everyone's responsibility to help stop FGM, regardless of where they come from.

We need decision makers in my country to raise public awareness and make full use of existing anti-FGM legislation. The *Prohibition of Female Genital Mutilation Act,* which became law in Uganda in March 2010, bans all types of FGM. The law, which must now be enforced, addresses the prosecution of promoters and cutters, and protects girls and women.

MALAWI

The practice of FGM, although it undoubtedly happens in some places, is very secret. Few facts are established about it and there is no known legislation to prevent it. Ms M was born in Malawi where, she stresses, children were obliged to follow the commands of their parents without question. It was at the age of ten that she underwent female genital mutilation, in a very rural part of the Malawi. Ms M moved to the UK in 2004. This is the first time she has chosen to campaign against FGM.

Ms M

Female genital mutilation was a practice in my culture when I was growing up, but I didn't know it as that term until into my adult years.

I was born in Malawi and lived in the rural area, in a village far away from civilisation. I grew up with all my family but my dad had to travel to Zambia, South Africa and some other countries in the region in search of work in the mines, and would return home maybe twice in a year. It was the norm back then for most families to be in this situation.

As my dad was away my brothers and I would help out my mum in the fields, fetching firewood, collecting water from the river, going to the river to do laundry and any other work that needed to be done. It was never easy as I grew up so fast; and yet I was young and life carried on. We would wake up early, do the fire and help out with all the house chores before going to school. At times all of us would also go and help out other families in the fields so that we could have some food on the table.

We had values instilled while we were young and carried on into adulthood, manners and traditions were taught all the time and up to now I still find it difficult not to curtsy for people in authority.

We never disobeyed, loyalty and openness was instilled and I would never hide any information from my family. I would attend traditional ceremonies in the village and my mum told me what it was all about, even though I did not understand some of these things.

As my dad was away my uncle was the father figure to my family, even though no one liked him. My dad was often away and sent him money to give us, but he never did. My mum tried her level best to provide the little that she could get. I have always wondered if my dad had another family somewhere else, as many men did.

I remember very well when I was ten years old my mum telling me I was going to be a grown up woman, she started telling me more and more each time we went for traditional ceremonies in the village. She would at times send me to stay with my aunt, who told me a lot of things, some of which had no meaning to me as I was just a young, pretty and beautiful innocent girl growing up.

My aunt also told me before she passed away that my dad and uncle wanted me to be a housewife and stay with someone and have babies. True to her story my dad had met this man in South Africa, where they worked in the mines together, and as is the tradition they arranged it all without my knowledge.

When I asked my mum all she said was that it was our tradition and culture and I should listen to elders. If I had had somewhere to run to I would have ran as fast and as far away as I could, but I had nowhere to go and I was scared and terrified each time I saw my uncle. I hated him and never wanted to see him. To this day I cannot stand him. He is non-existent to me. He used to keep an eye on me at all times. He would tell my mum that soon I was going to be a big woman and have a family.

I could not understand all this. I was young and my main intentions were to go to school and look after my mum and have a good job. Back then, a lot of our needs were difficult to meet, let alone schooling. I did go to school, but it was under a tree and I had to walk long distances, which was so tiring and never ending.

In 1979, when I was 13 or 14 years old, an elderly woman came and took me away. My mum was there but she could not protect me. I was taken in the middle of the night and stayed away from my family for close to two to three months with other girls of my age from my village, living in makeshift mud huts.

We were taught about 'being a woman' and I went through FGM (as it is known in today's world).

What I went through was painful, nasty, unbearable and sick.

I could not even walk for days as my body was all in pain and very sore. At that time it was normal for these older women to lecture and do all sorts of things in preparing us into womanhood. I was crying day and night for my mum.

After probably two and half months in the bush, far away from home, the whole camp was pulled down and we went back into our normal lives. When I was in the village I was meant to behave normally, never say anything about what happened when I was away as it was considered a taboo. I got so distanced from my brothers, I never want to see them. They knew all that I went through and they even knew the person who was going to be paired with me.

I still remember all the details, but I never discussed it with anyone, not even my family. I did intend to do this but circumstances beyond my control prevented me and in the end my mum and dad passed away with this topic still un-discussed. I do now have a son who is grown up, but he is resident in a different country from Malawi, so I haven't discussed it with him either.

I think it's a matter for the traditionally practising communities to address FGM themselves, with the assistance from the government and other agencies.

Although I've been away from the community for a long time, I presume that the secrecy continues although social media is now highlighting some of these issues. The fact that you are not meant to say anything is, I think, still the same.

Values and manners are instilled while young (maybe it's 'brainwashing' as I understand it in today's world?). It's taken me all these years to open up because culturally I was brought up being told to obey elders.

This whole topic makes me cry, to panic with anxiety, feel sick, upset, shaken and scared of people around me. Up to this day I have very bad terrible dreams and loads of nightmares that make me cry for help in my sleep.

I live in the UK now, and have worked in the Health and Social Care industry for the past ten years, but I am currently a stay-at-home partner. Until now I haven't been active in any campaigns against FGM; but then I had to open up and discuss things, when I was very down and low. I kept having nightmares and had a lot to consider about my life.

My GP has been a real help. I've had some sessions with a therapist and it's ongoing.

To stop FGM we will need to educate the communities that have these practices. I could have suggested campaigning in the village where I grew up, but I never want anything to do with it. I am not yet strong enough to face going there, especially as my parents are no longer alive.

FGM makes me sad. To eradicate FGM we must bring greater awareness to the public. Maybe this book could be translated into the languages of some communities in which these practices are very prevalent?

....

We shall meet other campaigners from or supporting the Sub-Saharan and Southern Africa movement in the chapters which follow, and you can read more news of the activists in this chapter on the Female Mutilation Worldwide website. The other African-heritage survivors and campaigners include Khadija Gbla, born in Gambia and now in Australia, Angela Peabody from Liberia and Barbara Mhangami Ruwende from Zimbabwe, and both now in the USA, and Valentina Acava Mmaka, who lived in South Africa and is now back in Italy.

Valentine Nkoyo and Esther Oenga, both born in Kenya, Virginia Kamara from South Africa, Comfort Ottah, Amanda Epe and Ms B (respectively, Nigerian and Yoruba heritage), Virginia Kamara, born in South Africa and Dr Phoebe Abe and

Sarah McCullock from Uganda, all now live in the UK.

It is the synergies between, and joint determination of, campaigners who remain in their native land and those who start new lives in other countries, that have revealed the extent of female genital mutilation as a global phenomenon. This global reach will be explored more in our next chapter, which focuses on Egypt, the Middle East and Southeast Asia.

CHAPTER 5:

Egypt, the Middle East &
Southeast Asia

This chapter examines female genital mutilation in Egypt, the Middle East and Southeast Asia. The geographical spread is wide – from north-eastern Africa to almost Australia – but one theme which seems to recur is the reluctance by the authorities (historically or currently) to acknowledge that female genital mutilation occurs, or is a problem.

We know that around ninety per cent of women in Egypt have experienced some sort of FGM, and that increasingly it is practised by medical personnel. It has been made illegal and there was a successful prosecution, on appeal, of a doctor recently, but the practice continues in many places.

Very little is currently known about the prevalence of FGM in the other countries considered here. Thanks to researchers, including the narrators in this book, new evidence is, however, coming to light which makes it clear FGM continues as a deeply embedded tradition in various parts of the Middle East and Southeast Asia. Our correspondents here share the results of their research and enquiries to date, and tell us about the various approaches which they have devised and adopted to counter this challenge.

OVERVIEW

Hannah Wettig is the Coordinator of the Stop FGM Middle East campaign by the Iraqi-German NGO WADI, which is based in Suleymania, Iraq and Frankfurt, Germany [Ch.8]. Research over the years has revealed that FGM occurs not only in the Middle East, but also across several parts of Asia. Hannah's remit with Stop FGM now also includes these areas as well as the campaign's original focus.

***

It was whilst in Egypt, in 1994, that I first heard about female genital mutilation. I was working as a journalist in the Middle East (and training to be an editor of a daily newspaper).

Later I became involved in development assistance, first as a speech writer and editor at the Ministry for Economic Cooperation and Development, then for an NGO supporting democracy activists in Syria. Since that time, I have become Coordinator of the Stop FGM Middle East campaign, based in Frankfurt, Germany.

Stop FGM Middle East is an initiative by WADI e.V. supported by Hivos, an international organisation that seeks new solutions to persistent global issues. WADI was founded in 1992 and is an Iraq-German non-profit association, which strives to empower people and strengthen human, especially women's, rights in the Middle East. The campaign Stop FGM Kurdistan is one of WADI's best-known programmes.

Our Stop FGM Middle East campaign started off as a research and information project. We collected all the evidence we could find on FGM in the Middle East and published it, making it known to journalists and the United Nations. Along the way, we stumbled upon evidence in India, Pakistan, Thailand, Malaysia, Sri Lanka, the Maldives, Brunei and the Philippines, none of which are part of the Middle East. We had known about FGM in Indonesia, but not how widespread the practice was in that part of Asia. So, since no one was making this knowledge public, we decided to widen the project's scope and include all of Asia where FGM exists.

We began by contacting activists from several effected countries in Asia. We invited them to a conference and started to build a network reaching from the Arabian Peninsula to Malaysia and Indonesia.

One of our campaign's focal points since the start has been religion. While FGM is not related to religion everywhere, all the evidence in Asia points to a strong connection between Islam and FGM. In communities where FGM is practiced, a mix of motivations ranging from myths to preserving a girl's chastity to religion may be found, but the one reason which often keeps them from stopping it often turns out to be religion.

We realised early on that it is essential to find religious leaders who correct the assumption of FGM as an Islamic duty or recommended practice. Likewise, we support local campaigns where activists in the respective countries are ready for it.

For a number of countries we still lack reliable evidence. If people make information about FGM in Asian countries known, this is always helpful. Please write about it on your blog or if you are a journalist or researcher try to find out more.

There is still a hesitance to name religion as one motivation behind FGM. We have started to do so for Asia and we found that activists are very grateful for our openness, because without addressing this topic there will be no progress in eradicating FGM in their countries.

While many communities in Africa, like in Ghana or Burkina Faso, Christians and Jews in Ethiopia or Egypt practice FGM for non-religious reasons, in other places you have a similar situation as in Asia. Parts of the religious community or even the dominant law school (Islamic legal code), as in Somalia, promote FGM.

We believe this may be true for some parts of Africa as well, where religion plays an important role as a motivation, especially in Egypt, Somalia and Sudan, but probably also other places where I shouldn't allow myself an opinion because I know too little about them. (I am an Arabist and have lived in Egypt and visited Sudan, so I have some idea about the aforementioned.)

In the Sunni Shafi'i law school, female circumcision is an obligation. This cannot be ignored, because people will simply not listen to health reasons when their religion tells them otherwise. They will ask: 'How can my religion tell me to do something which is unhealthy?'

In contrast with Western people, who might answer, 'Maybe there is something wrong with my religion', most people in the Arab world will say, 'People who say FGM is harmful must be lying and they are trying to tarnish my religion.'

The only way not to offend religion and still talk about FGM is to tackle the issue and work with religious leaders, as we do in Iraq and Iran. In Egypt this has been done, but only official religious leaders connected to the regime have taken a stand against FGM. We probably also need to take this approach to the community level, to the Sheikhs in the villages.

From a different angle, genital cosmetic surgery and male circumcision are often discussed alongside FGM. However, they need to be treated differently even if debate is certainly necessary about these practices.

Concerning cosmetic genital surgery, I think it is a problematic trend that women (and men) want their bodies to be as perfect and smooth as possible. However, it is a completely different topic from FGM. It's a feminist issue in the countries where this trend exists. It's something to talk about.

Cosmetic genital surgery, however, is not child abuse, not a human rights issue and ultimately it is the decision of those women and men who would like to alter their bodies. They are grown-ups and they live in countries where one can expect adults to take informed free-will decisions.

This type of elective surgery is closer to risky behaviour like mountain climbing, war reporting or smoking. It cannot be compared with mutilating girls or requiring adult women before marriage to be cut.

Where there are complications, male circumcision (male genital mutilation) must be considered alongside FGM but, we need to see more reliable studies. Male circumcision can be harmful, but I don't know of any studies which differentiate between methods, so I also don't know if the complications come with all methods.

Male circumcision is however much more religiously required in some parts of the world than is FGM, and it is a particularly sensitive issue in Germany. Discussing this topic is now beginning in the respective communities and this is the place where it should start. It is a good thing that there is a movement on this issue in the USA, where it is not necessarily connected to religion. Hopefully that debate will gain momentum.

In our work on FGM we have supported studies in Oman and Iran and are working on a research tool kit and manual for small-scale studies, which can be conducted by activists themselves. We also support a project in Iran, an information campaign through lectures and training for housewives and parents in the province of Kermanshah.

In April (2015) one of our partner project coordinators in Iran added to his information campaign a couple and group therapy for FGM victims. This will be a pilot project as part of our new campaigning aim: to target men.

....

EGYPT

Mawaheb El-Mouelhy is an obstetrician and expert in public health (population and reproductive health) with many years' experience of working in her homeland of Egypt and elsewhere. The treatment and cessation of female genital mutilation has been a major focus of her work.

***

I have been a reproductive health provider for more than thirty years; I am also a feminist and concerned about women's rights.

In the late 1970s I worked in England, where I delivered Sudanese and African women, most of whom were circumcised or infibulated. That was what first raised my interest in female genital mutilation. Some of those women asked to be reinfibulated after extensive episiotomies and some of them had to deliver by Caesarian section because of the extensive mutilation.

I have worked as a clinician in Egypt, UK, Saudi Arabia and the United Arab Emirates. When I came back to Egypt and started working in a clinic in a disadvantaged area of Cairo, I noticed that the majority of my clients were circumcised, although not the same degree as the Sudanese and Africans. The type of FGM performed in my country is usually Types 1 or 2, which do not usually require cosmetic surgery, not the extensive type of infibulation, Type 3.

From that time onwards I have conducted research, raised awareness and advocated to stop FGM as well as other traditional harmful practices such as child marriage and violence against women. Being a doctor, people listen to you carefully and trust what you say, which has helped me a lot during campaigns.

The NGO I worked for on my return to Egypt, the Cairo Family Planning Association, was a pioneering organisation in that field. Its volunteers have spoken against FGM since the 1970s, when it was embarrassing or shameful to talk about it in public. They have continued to raise awareness about this harmful tradition ever since then.

Immediately after the International Conference on Population and Development (ICPD) in 1994, a task force was established in Egypt involving NGOs against FGM, individuals and experts interested in this issue, and some donors. I was a member of this task force. We succeeded in recruiting officials from the Ministry of Health and the National Council for Childhood and Motherhood to our cause, and pushed the topic up the national agenda as a priority.

I see many circumcised women in my clinic. Years ago, traditional birth attendants used to perform FGM, unfortunately now doctors are more and more involved. Because of governmental and non- governmental campaigns and efforts, along with media involvement, the ice was broken and it became easier for people to discuss FGM and to ask questions.

Those efforts resulted in a decree by the Ministry of Health forbidding doctors to perform FGM in 2007. Then the medical syndicate announced a statement against it, and in 2008 the Egyptian Parliament passed a law criminalising FGM. In 2014 a doctor who performed fatal FGM on a child was eventually given a custodial sentence.

Changing a practice that has been going on for hundreds of years is not easy, especially when people think it as is related to tradition and/or religion. The media are very important. Doctors and religious leaders can play a crucial role in supporting our efforts.

Education, especially for women, is important. The less educated women are, the more likely they are to have their daughters circumcised. Talking to men is also important. Although FGM is usually the mother's or grandmother's decision, it is the man who pays for it.

People link FGM with sexual desire, not with sexual satisfaction. This perception has to be corrected in the mind of those people. In Egypt, the main 'reason' for performing FGM is to reduce girls' sexuality and consequently keep them chaste and virgin.

According to the *2014 Demographic and Health Survey*, the prevalence of FGM among the older women are more or less the same, while there is some evidence that it is coming down among younger women and girls. None of the female members of my family are circumcised but in my circle the maids, the cook, and the house porter's daughters are all circumcised.

Societies that stick to the tradition are the rural ones, especially in the south of Egypt (Upper Egypt). Other harmful traditional practices include child marriage and domestic violence against women and girls, and recently harassment has become a concern.

The extensive campaigns and efforts and the involvement of the media since the creation of the task force made it easy to speak about FGM in public. Then after the revolution of January 2011, and especially under the rule of the Muslim Brothers 2012/13, all these efforts stopped and the power of the radical religious leaders (who were pro FGM) had increased. That was an extremely difficult time for us as campaigners against harmful traditional practices including FGM.

Now we are back on track, supported by national and international organisations. I think we are doing well with decision makers. Current governmental bodies are more understanding, and international organisations (including UN) are supportive.

Something is however missing. We do not have centres or clinics to deal with victims of FGM who need medical, psychological or social support. In addition to the complications of FGM, sometimes even death, it seems that sexual problems are increasing as a result. Women are now less shy to discuss these problems. Some divorce cases arise as a result of the couple's sexual dissatisfaction.

I am getting older and I want to see the younger generation continuing our efforts relentlessly. My wish for the future is to see the prevalence of illiteracy among our women as 0 per cent; women's education will help reducing harmful traditional practices.

Male circumcision however is mentioned in our holy book. It is required by religion, so I would not deal with that.

People should support our work against FGM in any way they can, by writing, by funding efforts and activities in Africa, by being involved in campaigns.

The question about whether FGM and other harmful traditional practices have significant economic impact on our communities is a very interesting. I was in a meeting with the World Health Organisation two weeks ago discussing violence against women (VAW) and I asked the question: what is the economic impact of VAW?

I think we need research to respond to the question. When complications happen as a result of FGM, how much is the cost of the time of doctors, nurses, medicines, medical management, blood transfusion, police, lawyers, judges. What is the cost of death?

....

YEMEN

Almost a quarter of the adult female population in Yemen has experienced FGM, where legislation to outlaw the practise has recently started to be developed.

Karima Amin is originally from Yemen, where she underwent female genital mutilation at the age of seven. She moved to Virginia USA two years later, in 1996. Karima wants everyone to understand what FGM entails, why it is so damaging to girls' futures, and why it must be stopped.

***

I had female genital mutilation done to me in 1994 in Yemen, when I was seven years old. We would hear about it in the area where we lived and I knew girls who had gone through it, but my father always said that it would never happen to me.

Unfortunately my father passed away and shortly afterwards the women in the area convinced my mother to arrange FGM for me. I ran away the first couple of times that the man came to do it to me, but one day he came really early. Before I could get up, a lady with him grabbed me and sat on my stomach.

My mother was afraid of blood, so she left and I was all alone with the man and woman. The man told me he would punish me for all those times I ran away. He performed the worst type.

That man closed everything. I couldn't even pass water. He had to come back the next day to poke a hole so I could pee. Afterwards, urinating was hard and my sister had to pour water on me so I could do it. I couldn't move and my legs were wrapped together. I had to be helped getting up and it was very painful. I shall never forget the first time I had to urinate. The wounds were still new so it was burning and I cried. I was only seven.

There were no repercussions. The man who did it to me was paid and he went on with his life. My family never brought it up although it was so painful. I have told my mom it shouldn't have happened, and she just said, 'Everyone was doing it, so I allowed it.' Unfortunately because of my culture and how I was raised, getting help was not an option. It was like, 'It happened, get over it.' We are also Muslims so talking about the private parts is a no-no.

That was two decades ago, but it still affects me every day. I have trouble passing urine and psychologically it bothers me. I have nightmares sometimes and have a hard time sleeping. I always felt I am not complete as a woman because I don't have my clitoris.

I don't live in Yemen anymore so I can't say for sure whether FGM is becoming less common there. I would also say that FGM is too barbaric and extreme for people in the mainstream to talk openly; but for my own community, I want to see education about the consequences.

Tell everyone about the dangers, and that girls can suffer long-term effects, experience problems when they want to have babies, and even die. Just educate the people, especially in Yemen in the rural poor areas where it's a completely taboo subject.

Mothers need to understand that their daughters will not turn out 'bad' if they don't get circumcised. The women believe the girls will be 'whores' and we need to make them understand that's not true. FGM doesn't solve any problems. It causes much harm to girls psychologically.

Two years after my experience we moved to the USA. I haven't heard much about female genital mutilation in America, but I know it's becoming more common in the UK.

Unfortunately a lot of the mothers, especially Somalis in the USA, are told that because their daughters live in the west with non-Muslims, these girls will sleep around and bring the family into disrepute, so the mothers think FGM is their only hope of avoiding shame.

I do not as yet have a family of my own mainly because I've shunned getting close to men. I was afraid of being with them, so it affected my relationships too. The girls I know who had it done have pain during sex and can't feel anything. They removed my parts so I was very uncomfortable with getting married because I was afraid of letting anyone see. I felt deformed. It ruined my self-esteem and I have battled depression.

Nonetheless, I recently got married and my husband has been wonderful and very supportive about everything. Now I'm having infertility problems and my doctor said it could be related to FGM. Hopefully this will be a wake-up call and change the minds of those who are in favour of FGM.

Because of my Islamic religion, I don't have many options around infertility, since surrogacy is not allowed and adopting can be complicated. I will be trying IVF and see how that goes.

It's all about our culture. To stop FGM we need to help mothers understand that talking to their daughters about sex and other personal stuff is OK and nothing to be embarrassed about. There's a lot of shame about this because of our culture and traditions.

Discussing FGM also brings too much pain for the actual victims. I can't speak for everyone but I just never want to remember that fateful day. For many years I've remained silent because FGM was too painful to talk about, but I'm ready now. I feel like I have finally let it stop controlling me and I no longer need to run away from the subject. I hope no more girls go through this barbaric practice.

I never want another precious, innocent little girl to experience what I did. It's been almost 21 years and I'm still affected by it.

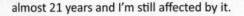

IRAQ

Maha Alsakban was born and lives in Iraq, where FGM occurs particularly on the Kurdistan border. Legislation again FGM has recently been introduced, but it continues. Mahais a doctor, a consultant paediatrician and civil society activist.

***

I am a consultant paediatrician specialising in neonates (newborn babies). My first experience of female genital mutilation therefore came some long while ago, around 1990, in the delivery rooms.

A patient in labour was having an obstructed delivery because of FGM, and the nurses had to open her external genitals by removing the sutures to assist her during child birth. I was in attendance to resuscitate the baby immediately after it was born, but I saw that the obstetric team had to re-suture the woman when the delivery was over.

This experience alerted me to the issues around FGM. I am a human rights activist and I campaign against FGM.

I have conducted interviews with women in practising communities, and I did a larger survey study targeting female in two provinces of Iraq, Wasit & Alqadssiya.

There are a lot of gender-related human rights issues where I live. These include honour killing, forced marriages, child and early (teenage) marriages, and for instance forcing young females to wear hijab (covering the hair and neck, the enforcement of which is done particularly by educational officials and teachers).

It is very difficult for people in traditional communities to speak out against these practices.

IRAN

Rayehe Mozafarian and Kameel Ahmady have both conducted research projects into the prevalence of female genital mutilation in Iran and made films about it.

Rayehe is Iranian, living there and researching FGM in her home country. Often a lone voice, she also speaks about FGM at conferences and on the radio and television. Kameel is a British-Iranian cultural anthropologist who for the past decade has been conducting academic research for an EndFGM project in his birthplace, Iranian Kurdistan, covering the three Kurdish western provinces of West Azerbaijan, Kermanshah, Kurdistan and the southern province of Hormozgan.

***

Rayehe Mozafarian

The first time I knew about female genital mutilation was when my mum gave me a book, *Desert Flower* by Waris Dirie, which had been translated into my own language, Persian. The book led me to ask whether FGM occurs in Iran, where I was born and live.

I started searching on Google but found only two or three reports of FGM, in Kurdish areas of Iran and a city in the south. That's when I decided to start my journeys of exploration. At the time, I was selecting a subject for my college thesis. Which subject better than FGM in Iran? I worked for three years, writing and collecting my data. After finishing my study I published it as a book entitled *Razor and Tradition*. That book was also published in Persian, but I translated some parts of it into English. These translated sections were included in the report by an Austrian NGO, Südwind, in 2014, *Violations of Girls' Rights: Child Marriage and FGM in the I.R. Iran*.

My friend and colleague Fatemeh Karimi has also written a book about these issues, *Tragedy of the Body, Violence against Women* (2010).

I studied demography and development in Shiraz University, Iran. I come from a privileged family and they encouraged me to develop my abilities and talents, but it is hard for ordinary people to work in fields such as FGM, because they need a salary. Fortunately, my situation enables me to devote my life on this subject and related women's issues, so I am a volunteer, sustained by my family, especially my mother.

I have made a film about FGM in Iran, and I attend conferences, give talks, write articles and use social media to tell people about FGM and why it must stop.

It is difficult to explain how I feel. Sometimes I am happy when I see the positive reaction of audiences and they want to help. At other times I can't control my anger because I know FGM is happening but everybody wants to convince me it was only in the past! But I will confront these limitations and blocks. I remind myself every time:

Even one victim is too many.

Internal and official Iranian media did not want to support me or talk about FGM, so I focussed on the Iranian media abroad and started writing for them. I also sent my book to the Iranian government for permission to publish it, but three times they refused. So I published it in France instead.

A year later, the government changed and Rouhani became president, so I resubmitted my book. Finally, in February 2015, I obtained permission to publish in Iran, and one of the official Iranian newspapers started to write about my book. Then I sent all my information and a lot of copies of my book to the related official and governmental organisations, to ensure they were aware that FGM is still happening.

We did not know the exact extent of FGM in Iran, or whether it is becoming less common, because there was no exact data before our efforts, but we are taking the first steps towards eradication, as people start hearing about FGM. Many people do not know it is done, and there are a lot of others who do know, but they do not want to talk about it and destroy their culture.

There are also other domestic violations like early and forced marriage, honour killings and female self-immolation. All traditionally practising communities make it difficult to speak out on these matters.

It is very difficult to work in the Middle East. I cannot invite another person to work with me under these conditions. I don't have permission to work in this area or any security.

Across Iran, EndFGM activists start alone as volunteers, doing field work. Why can't we develop training for these volunteers, providing opportunities to attend dedicated study courses and then go back to their society and work? Exactly as in Iraqi-Kurdistan we need to organise workshops, publish booklets and talk more and more with people at different levels, such as midwives, nurses, doctors, local leaders, religious leaders and others.

And just as in Africa, we need an Ambassador and a centre or organisation or institute in the Middle East and Asia for organizing and cooperating with governments and international organisations. In fact, we need this programme for the world not just for the Middle East.

I want to see demographic and epidemiological studies, open data and publishing, better legislation, education and women's empowerment, FGM-aware and skilled professionals, and scholarship to develop required skills (for psychologists, psychoanalysts, sociologists, gynaecologists, physicians, midwives, religious leaders, lawyers etc.). And there are also other harmful traditional practices (HTPs) for which professionals need training, e.g. FGM reconstructive and fistula surgery.

I discussed these harmful traditional practices and related issues in my work and I've translated articles written in other languages into Persian. I made a film about FGM, *Razor and Tradition*, and have written books (including one with the same name as the film) and reports on FGM and its eradication. These books have been published both in Iran and beyond its borders.

I also think male circumcision, which some people call MGM, is an issue to be considered at some point, but I do not want to mix these two subjects. My concern is focussed on female genital mutilation.

We in the Middle East need a permanent research centre to study the history and culture of mutilation in all its forms, as punishment, as tradition, as treatment.

We also need formal representation on FGM to the UN from the Middle East. The World, UNICEF and the UN do not acknowledge that FGM is an Asian and Middle Eastern problem too. If we cannot reach our goals ourselves, which organisation will assume this responsibility, whilst we do not have any international or public support, and our government remains in denial? How much we can tolerate?

UNICEF has listed 29 countries where FGM continues, but there are ten or more Asian and Middle Eastern countries still waiting to be added!

***

Kameel Ahmady

In 2005 I returned from Europe to my birthplace, Iranian Kurdistan after an absence of many years, to find out more about FGM. I had been working in Africa with humanitarian relief NGOs and had observed United Nations projects and UNICEF combating FGM in counties like Somalia, Kenya and Sudan.

Remembering vaguely from my childhood 35 years ago that female genital mutilation existed in some parts of Iranian Kurdistan, I conducted preliminary research, starting with my own family and close relatives, and found much shocking evidence that FGM has long existed in areas of Mukriyan including my very own family. My sisters, mother and grandmothers had all been circumcised.

I then made a film, *In the Name of Tradition*, about FGM in that region of Iran. This anthropological documentary contains footage and a total of about nine thousand interviews from remote locations in West Azerbaijan, Kurdistan, Kermanshah and Hormozgan province, including islands such as Qeshm, Hormuz and Kish.

With help from a number of female research assistants, I interviewed local women and women circumcisers ('bibis', the professional cutters) and also sought the opinion of local men, medical staff and clerics in these less accessible and reported rural areas of Iran.

Overall, the initial fact-finding, fieldwork, training and eradication programmes continued from 2005 to 2014. I have been managing the study.

After the initial pilot, we decided the research would focus on rural locations rather than urban and cosmopolitan areas. The reasons for this decision included lack of funding, available legal authorisations and evidence from our preliminary research that FGM is much less likely to happen in urban areas these days.

We therefore first visited randomly selected villages in preselected parts of the country and then, years later, implemented more comprehensive targeted village by village data collections, training and pilot projects.

Our investigations revealed that Hormozgan province has the highest rate of FGM in Iran. We also explored whether other regions were affected by FGM. The study revealed that although Sunni (Shafi sect) communities – thought to be most likely to practise FGM – exist in some other provinces, no evidence of FGM could be found. FGM appears to be concentrated in the Hormozgan province's southern regions and islands.

In addition to the Sunni population, FGM was also found in women in their fifties or older among Shia Kurds, but it seems no young girls have been circumcised, so the tradition of FGM has disappeared in most of these communities. However, some Shia from the south still practise FGM alongside Sunnis.

Our pilot programme to combat FGM involved diversified approaches and included different phases, strategies methods, approaches and training manuals according to local sensitivities and languages.

We held face-to-face meetings with community stakeholders and awareness-raising sessions, mainly with young women and using a range of methods to outline the dangers of FGM for women health and even lives.

We also engaged with groups of men in mosques, on the doorstep and in many public places. Lobbying was conducted with community leaders and most importantly with clerics (both men and women of the Sufi Mevlevi order in the south of Iran, who have an ancient tradition of whirling dances) as well local sheikhs. We sought their support to ban FGM and asked them to issue local fatwas to that effect.

The same villages were visited again a year later to assess the success and impact of the pilot programmes. Our findings are as follows:

- The role of government in combatting FGM is critically important.
- National interventions in education and health programmes are necessary to protect girls and disseminate messages about ending FGM.
- We need bespoke education programmes, which accommodate local cultural understandings.
- Many religious and cultural traditionalists of influence in Kurdish society support FGM. The task of opposing it is difficult and sometimes perilous.
- Health providers have significant capacity to take the End FGM message to the wider population of well women, in addition to those already with problems.
- The potential of the conventional media to change attitudes and stop FGM is huge.
- Social media can reach young people and encourage them to connect with wider global communities.
- There is currently a dearth of empirical information about FGM, and about the effectiveness of eradication programmes, in Iran. Funding for such research is required.

- In campaigning against FGM it must be remembered that some women and girls have already undergone it. Their needs must be met in culturally sensitive ways.

The incidence of FGM in affected areas of Iran has fallen every year during our study. We attribute this change in part to our specific programme, and also to increasing modernity, the lack of new bibis to replace older excisers, a lack of willingness by girls now to undergo FGM, overall higher levels of education, and the impact of the media. It is helpful that some influential local clerics have also endorsed the End FGM message.

Whilst male circumcision is also potentially harmful, that issue is yet to be considered. There is however a greater willingness in communities now to discuss matters such as FGM, and younger people are challenging their elders' views on it.

I hope to launch my book about this research, along with a short documentary, in Iran and London, on the International Day Against Child Violence, 4 June, 2015.

....

PAKISTAN

FGM is known to occur in a few areas of Pakistan, especially the Dahwoodi Bohra community. The national prevalence overall may be around 10 per cent.

Qamar Nassem was born into a conservative family in Peshawar, Pakistan, where the women had no status and were unable to make choices for themselves. Even women's personal health matters were, he observed, decided by men. Concerned about this situation, in 1999 Qamar formed a not-for-profit organisation, *Blue Veins*, to raise awareness of breast cancer in his region of the country. Since then the remit of this charity has since expanded enormously, to include many other issues (including female genital mutilation). The challenges of working in a society where discussion of sexuality or any other matter related to women is almost taboo, remain immense, and sometimes personally perilous.

***

Most people around the world are unaware that the brutal practice of female genital mutilation exists in Pakistan, where it is commonly known as a *female khatna*. Though FGM takes place, the practice is hidden, hardly ever spoken of, barely acknowledged. The country, for instance, is considered to be 'free' of FGM, like a number of other Muslim-majority countries in the region.

FGM is rarely known in Pakistan, except in Sindh and the Bohra and Sheedi communities, where some people reason that FGM is part of their culture, in a similar way to paying dowry or naming children after relatives.

There are roughly one hundred thousand Bohra Muslims in the country, mostly in the southern regions of Pakistan, such as Sindh. In recent years, due to a rise in strict sect religious compliance by the Bohra Muslims, the practice of FGM has increased. Unless the Bohra chief, known as Dai, issues a decree to forbid the act, the practice will remain firmly rooted in the people's culture and will continue to be practiced.

50 to 60 per cent of Bohra women undergo circumcision, involving usually a symbolic snipping of the clitoris. In the past there was more aggressive mutilation, and I think 80 to 90 per cent of women suffered it. More awareness has helped reduce the invasiveness of the practice.

The ethnic Sheedi Muslim community of Pakistan, considered to be of Arab-African origin, also practice FGM. The Sheedi community, which numbers several thousand, came to the country originally as slaves during the nineteenth and twentieth centuries, and is also based primarily in Sindh. There has been little research on the practice among these groups.

The practice of FGM is also found in Muslim communities near Pakistan's Iran-Baluchistan border and occasionally for religious reasons in isolated families all over Pakistan, but the incidence of this practice overall is very low and no data is available or collected to gauge its scale.

Nonetheless, FGM remains a challenge for us in Pakistan. My organisation, Blue Veins, an emerging group of activists embracing the motto 'Awareness, Action and Advocacy', is working to stop FGM and other practices which prevent women from being the equal of men.

On a basic level, we have had to confront the idea that education is only for boys. Schools have been attacked by ultra-conservative groups and we have had to rebuild them. But we also identify these challenges as damaging men as well as women. For instance, preventing women from seeking medical advice for health issues helps no-one.

We seek to help men move away from violence and harassing girls, we stress that questions of 'family honour' will not be resolved by harming someone and we encourage people to think about matters such as sex and gender relationships, which are not part of normal discourse in the contexts of tribal norms and values. We try to have dialogue with everyone, and so for instance we involve men by speaking to individuals at the *hurja* (local community gatherings).

Male chauvinism is a cocoon from which men must emerge. Everyone is happier when girls and boys, men and women, coexist in peace. This is not comfortable or easy work; but we handle our programmes carefully.

Progress is however slow. Many challenges remain, nor is it 'just' the young women of Pakistan who are subjected to FGM in my country.

In the UK young British girls of Pakistani heritage pack their best clothes and favourite treasures, excited at the thought of a long visit to see their relatives, usually in the Bohra or Sheedi communities of Pakistan. These little girls don't know that, when they arrive, the plan is for them to undergo female genital mutilation.

. . . .

MALAYSIA

It is likely that a large majority of the female population in Malaysia has undergone FGM. There is no noted legislation against it. **Ms C** was born and lives in Malaysia. She studied Sociology and Anthropology at university. Ms C has worked for a women's rights NGO since 2000, which was when she first encountered reports of female genital mutilation. More recently she realised that, as a baby, she had herself undergone FGM.

***

I have been working for a Malaysian organisation concerned with women's rights since 2000, and I become aware of FGM in my country only after reading news reports and research work about it.

I have never witnessed any FGM being done to anyone in my entire life. Mothers and grandmas normally arrange for it to be done when baby girls are still small, from one to six months old, so that they won't know about the pain and remember it. Until recently the procedure was carried out by traditional midwives, and now more doctors are doing it.

I don't recall anything about my own FGM. I knew about it when I asked my mother. Because of the age when it is done, if you don't ask, you will never know.

FGM is not considered a big issue in my country. It was nothing unusual for me until recently. I don't know of a single incident when girls or women have been upset about going through FGM. I only started to take FGM seriously quite recently, although I have been aware of the African practice way back since 2000.

I don't think my family oppose FGM; they are accustomed to it. They do FGM to their daughters and it has always been associated with religious requirements. My country doesn't call it female genital mutilation', but instead it's called FC (female circumcision). Types I, II and IV are practised here in Malaysia, but we don't have full infibulation.

The organisation I am attached to aims to 'promote an understanding of Islam that recognises the principles of justice, equality, freedom and dignity within a democratic state'. People are always asking us for a statement and comment when it comes to issues around FC.

The institutions in Malaysia involved with FC matters are the *National Fatwa Council* (which released a fatwa – a religious decree - saying that FC is compulsory for all Muslim girls/women), the Ministry of Health (for medicalizing FC now, although they know there is no medical benefit behind FC) and women's rights groups which put pressure on agencies which condone FC.

It bothers me when Muslims particularly practice FC, as if it is a religious call, which is not. Jews, Christians and other religions have practised FC before Islam came. It is an old traditional practice.

FC is predominantly practiced by the Muslim community here. According to a research done by Dr Maznah Dahlui from the University of Malaya in collaboration with WHO, 93 per cent of Muslim girls in this country have undergone FC.

The practice is not getting any less common and unfortunately Muslim doctors also condone it, because people believe FGM is a religious requirement. From my study, I could not find a single verse promulgating FGM in the Holy Quran. References can only be found in Hadiths, which are collections of reports of the teachings, deeds and sayings of the Prophet Muhammad s.a.w. (PBUH).

Hadiths are classified into four types – Sahih (sound), Hasan (good), Da`if (weak) or Maudu` (fabricated, forged). Many hadiths condoning FGM are classified as weak, narrated by the person who either doesn't have a strong (authenticated / corroborated) account, or isn't virtuous. Prophet Muhammad did not do any circumcision to any of his daughters.

Traditionally practising communities in Malaysia are open about FGM but most people would oppose the idea that their daughters should not be circumcised. They believe any effort to reform traditional practices is a Western agenda.

I want everyone to understand about FGM:
- FGM is not to do with Islam, other religions had practiced FGM way before Islam came.
- Not a single verse from the Holy Quran condones FGM, the practise derives from weak Hadith.
- FGM is a form of violence against women and a violation of children's rights.
- No medical benefit derives from FGM.
- FGM is a form of control over women's bodies, and a sign of deep-rooted patriarchy.

My message to decision makers in Malaysia is:

- National Fatwa Council – abolish the fatwa stating that FC is compulsory for Muslim girls.
- Ministry of Health – punish doctors who choose to do FC, and criminalise FGM.

It would be good to know more about reconstructive surgery for FGM and for fistula. FGM should be completely abolished; international pressure on the ruling government is needed to stop FGM.

We are aware that eradicating FGM will have economic impacts on the traditional midwives and doctors who practice it. This service is not free and the fee is around RM 80–300 (£ 15–55 / 21–77 / $ 22–84) per 'package'. If performed by midwives, the package may also include ear piercing for babies and post-natal massage for mothers.

....

INDONESIA

A large majority of women in Indonesia are thought to have undergone FGM. There is legislation against it, but, following another directive that it should be performed, medicalisation has probably actually increased the incidence of the practice.

Rena Herdiyani is an Indonesian citizen working for a women's rights organisation, Kalyanamitra, based in Jakarta. She became aware of female genital mutilation in her country in 2005, when some women's groups began to lobby the Indonesian government to ban the medicalisation of FGM.

***

I was born in Indonesia and now work for Kalyanamitra, a women's rights non-profit organisation (NGO) established in 1985 and based in Jakarta. It was only in 2005 that I first heard about FGM.

Kalyanamitra is involved in campaigns to stop FGM. We use many different ways to do this such as lobbying, discussions and seminars, documentary films and working with international organisations like Terre Des Femmes (in Germany), Amnesty International and Equality Now UK.

We also report the facts about FGM in Indonesia via United Nations Human Rights mechanisms such as the *Convention on the Elimination of All Forms of Discrimination against Women* (CEDAW), the *International Covenant on Civil and Political Rights* (ICCPR), the *Universal Periodic Review* (UPR*), International Covenant on Economic, Social and*

Cultural Rights (ICESCR) and the *United Nations Human Rights Special Rapporteur.*

In my work with Kalyanamitra I am trying to get support to help us develop a creative digital campaign to stop FGM, using IT and social media to raise public awareness in Indonesia. Mainstream society should be involved actively in the campaigns to stop FGM; we want to build a wide consensus of public opinion against it.

We also need effective strategies for eradicating FGM in practising communities (urban, poor and rural communities). I think the most effective methods are community discussions, building networking with religious and community leaders, and collaboration with media (local radio, TV, newspapers) to campaign on stopping FGM. I don't, however, have any definitive facts on whether FGM is now becoming less common.

People in the affected communities still find it difficult to speak out because they are afraid to be different from the majority who agree with FGM on behalf of religion and culture. They think there is no negative impact if they perform FGM because most of them are not cutting into the female genitals. Male circumcision or male genital mutilation (MGM) could be used as a material discussion/campaign alongside of FGM from a health perspective, when we discuss the issues with doctors, midwives and traditional practitioners.

Although FGM practices in Indonesia have a lesser impact on survivors than FGM practices in Africa (the 'cutting' is less invasive here), FGM is still violence against women and there is no benefit for women's health.

In Indonesia, political pressure is exerted on the government by the Indonesian Ulema Council - Indonesia's top Muslim clerical body, which acts as an interface between the Indonesian government, which is secular, and the Islamic community – to maintain the practice of FGM. I need help from progressive Islamic jourists to influence the mindset of the Indonesian Ulema Council, who remain conservative on the issue of FGM.

Conservative religious interpretation is a big barrier to advocacy against FGM and how to change people's mindsets, even though FGM is not a required Islamic religious practice. I have a wish that Indonesia will be free from any form of FGM, and that we will have clear regulation to ban it. We must campaign against FGM in my country via social media and by writing about FGM in Indonesia for the international media.

FGM has a significant economic impact on my country because in certain ethnic groups in Indonesia, such as the Makassar, they have parties and invite people to celebrate when their girls are circumcised, even when they come from poor families.

My message to decision makers in Indonesia is simple. Ban FGM in Indonesia, right now.

. . . .

Thanks to researchers and campaigners like those above, our knowledge of FGM in Egypt, the Middle East and Southeast Asia is extending rapidly. You can check out developments in their work on the Female Mutilation Worldwide website, which will carry reports of the work and progress of campaigners, as the authorities in these regions recognise more fully the need for action. In parallel, awareness of the global extent of FGM is now being heightened by lobbies and campaigns in various parts of the Western world, including in Australia, our next port of call.

CHAPTER 6:

Australia

This Chapter comprises essentially a case study of one national anti-female genital mutilation organisation. Campaigns to eradicate female genital mutilation do not arise from nowhere. The No FGM Australia movement, which formalised only quite recently, illustrates some of the complexities of developing such a campaign.

Our Australian contributors are all connected through their involvement in *No FGM Australia*. Three of them – Paula Ferrari, the founder, Khadija Glba (one of the few survivors now in Australia to speak out) and Sybil Williams – are Directors of the organisation. Ms L is a volunteer supporter of the campaign. All hold Australian citizenship. Paula is by profession a teacher and speech pathologist, Khadija is studying law, Sybil is a consultant communications specialist, and Ms L, a lawyer.

THE SURVIVOR

Khadija Gbla was born in Sierra Leone, but in 2001, aged 13, she and her family fled to Australia after attaining refugee status via the United Nation's Refugee Program. Before that, they had sought refuge in Gambia from more than a decade of civil war in Sierra Leone. It was in Gambia, when she was nine, that Khadija underwent female genital mutilation. One of the few survivors in Australia who speak out against FGM, Khadija is now a director of the not-for-profit organisation No FGM Australia.

***

My experience of female genital mutilation is still something which my mother and I rarely discuss. To live in peace we need to avoid the subject. She still does not seem to perceive any need to apologise for what she did. Any discussion about FGM is, she insists, shameful and inappropriate.

But my choice has been to beat the shame, to banish it by talking to everyone and telling them that FGM is massively wrong, and must stop. Now. I am an African Australian in a society where women's entitlement to bodily integrity and to normal sexual pleasure is acknowledged. FGM invaded my most sacred place. It robbed me of something very precious. A part of me died that day when I was forced brutally to endure female genital mutilation.

My mother and others in our community of her generation believe there is a non-negotiable obligation on mothers from our homeland, Sierra Leone, to ensure that daughters go through Bondo as a rite of passage before they reach maturity. They are convinced FGM is required for self-control, and that discussion of it is shameful.

'Bondo' is the name used in Sierra Leone to refer to FGM, and is also the name of the women's secret society, like the 'Sande', which conducts this initiation. The society has huge influence in Sierra Leone and across much of West Africa. From my mother's perspective, any female who has not undergone FGM, whatever her age, is not clean and will be ruled by her sexual urges.

My mother was effectively compelled by the tradition of Bondo to be actively involved in my so-called 'empowerment' at the age of nine - via the brutal removal, without anaesthetic and in a grossly unhygienic setting, of most of my external genitalia. She believed, and continues to believe, that this cruel act was inescapably necessary to be certain that later on I wouldn't as a teenager 'go around having sex with everybody like women who haven't had circumcision', and so I would be considered 'clean'.

My mother and almost everyone else in Sierra Leone of her generation believes that clitoridectomy is 'empowering'. She says that, without a clitoris, women can actually manage to refuse sex with their husbands if there is a marital dispute; it is her belief that ensuring daughters have what she calls 'circumcision' is a mother's duty, doing the child a favour.

I was born in Freetown, Sierra Leone in 1988. My grandfather was a chief with three wives and considerable influence; but when I was three years old, in 1990, civil war broke out and our social visibility placed us in great danger. People were trying to kill us, bombs were dropping, women were being targeted for unbelievable atrocities, butchered, raped and sold into slavery. We fled, eventually ending up in Gambia, lucky to escape with our lives.

Then, a while after we arrived in Gambia, when I was nine years old, my mother applied for refugee status. We were delighted when our application was eventually accepted, and we learned that we were going to Australia, which we knew was comfortingly far away, at the 'end of the world'.

But before we departed for our new life my mother and another elder woman took me and my sister on what she called a holiday, something we never did. We drove for hours through the Gambian bush and eventually we arrived in a very remote area where there were just two little huts. Waiting for us was a very old, very scary lady who spoke with my mother and then went back inside one of the huts.

By this time I was really anxious about what was going on, but as an African child you don't question your parents, you just say 'Yes, ma'am' and 'Yes, sir'.

A few minutes later the old lady reappeared, holding a very rusty, very dirty short knife. She went into the other hut, and my mother forced me to follow her. Within seconds my clothes had been removed and I was pinned to the ground. I thought I was going to be slaughtered there and then, but instead the old lady slid down my body and started to use her blunt, rusty old knife to hack off my clitoris and labia.

I struggled against my mother as hard as I could, but to no avail, and I screamed in agony, but no-one came to my rescue, and the old woman just continued cutting into me inch by inch. Eventually she managed to saw my clitoris and labia off completely, then she threw away my hacked off flesh as though it was the most disgusting thing she had ever seen. The job done, she just got up and walked away, leaving me bleeding, in agony and, most of all, confused about what had just happened.

The trauma of that day, and of what my mother permitted to happen to me will stay with me forever.

Afterwards I bled for weeks. I was taken to a friend's house for a while to recover. I was made to sit frequently in a tub of disinfectant, apparently because this was believed to help with the pain. Walking was a nightmare, as though I had something stuck between our legs, for weeks and weeks.

Later, when my periods started; and so did my personal hell. Each month the bleeding went on for days and days, and we had to call out the ambulance to take me for morphine shots to subdue the pain.

But unlike many girls, I didn't actually die as a result of this brutality – though I was fearful for my life again much later on, because of FGM, when I went into labour with my beautiful (and, thankfully, thriving) baby son.

When we first arrived in Australia I was the only black child in my (girls') school. I was sick all the time (because of the FGM, though I didn't know that then) and bullied. Australia didn't feel like the land of happy opportunity that I had expected, so after a while I decided to stop focussing on the negatives and find something positive to do.

I volunteered for an organisation called Women's Health Statewide and became involved in their FGM programme. I ran sessions for doctors and nurses about what FGM entails, explaining that it still happens because people believe women must be virgins and 'pure' right up until they marry. That way, as marketable commodities, they will attract a good bride price (dowry). I also explained that, most of all, FGM is a way to control women's sexuality.

It was still two months before, one day looking at diagrams of the types of FGM after a WHS session, it suddenly hit me that FGM had happened to me, personally.

Within seconds I was back in the bush, the old lady bearing down on me with her knife. I had been so traumatised by FGM that until that moment I'd blanked it out, forgotten about it completely.

I went home that night and asked my mother why she had made me undergo FGM. She said it wasn't FGM, it was 'just circumcision, a favour' which was to keep me from being 'itchy down there'. As a teenager who had read a lot in girls' magazines about women's naughty bits, I wondered if I was talking to an alien, because it sounded like my mother came from another planet.

Right now there are a few cases of alleged FGM going through the Australian courts. Tragically, girls in Australia are *not* yet safe from FGM.

That's why I started an e-petition in Australia, demanding that Prime Minister Tony Abbott and the Minister for Women Michaelia Cash act to protect Australian girls from FGM. I want them to convene a cross-ministerial meeting by the end of 2015 to plan and align strategies to eliminate this brutal practice in Australia.

We must also make full use of compelling, heart-breaking films and documentaries such as Equality Now's *Africa Rising*, which The *Sydney Feminists* and *No FGM Australia* collaboratively screened in 2014.

People in Australia still do not really understand how serious the FGM problem is; but in fact there are two things which must be done. The first thing is to develop effective prevention strategies, as our e-petition asks. Further, these preventative interventions must address both FGM and other traditional practices that harm women and children.

The second required action is to take seriously the need to provide for girls and women who, like me, have already undergone FGM. FGM does long-lasting harm to physical health and to psychological well-being.

Moving forward from the repercussions of FGM is not easy; affected individuals need help to learn how to manage, even though in reality the fact of FGM will never actually go away.

I will continue campaigning for however long it takes, addressing the challenges which confront immigrants and refugees as they arrive in Australia, speaking out at every opportunity against all forms of violence against women and girls, and working with No FGM Australia to eradicate FGM as soon as we possibly can.

I have been fighting against genital torture since I was 13, half a lifetime ago. I have experienced all these problems and tribulations at first hand. I am determined also to contribute to their solutions.

***

Paula Ferrari is Australian, living in Melbourne. Trained as a teacher and speech pathologist, she in now Managing Director of No FGM Australia, an organisation which she founded and on which she collaborates with her co-directors, Khadija Gbla and Sybil Williams. Like many other current activists, Paula first learnt of FGM whilst a student, believing it then to be a matter of history, rather than of contemporary concern.

I am a mother of three and a health professional and registered primary school teacher in Victoria, Australia.

I first encountered FGM in the 1990s, when I read Alice Walker's pivotal book, *Possessing the Secret of Joy*. As a sexually aware young woman, I was quite horrified at the thought of mutilating the sexual organs of women, apparently to control and prevent them experiencing sexual pleasure. What seemed even more perverse to me was that girls were convinced mutilation was somehow an honour, so they volunteered for FGM, only discovering too late what it really meant.

Back then I was not in a position to 'do' anything about what I had just learnt and anyway I thought it was an ancient practice, no longer happening in these modern times, especially not in Australia.

All teachers and health professionals are required by law to report any child abuse, physical, emotional or sexual. During my professional training however I was never, ever made aware of female genital mutilation as one possible sort of abuse.

Then in 2012, I was sent a petition at random by a friend asking for governments to 'Stop FGM'. Seeing the photo of a little girl, perhaps aged six or seven, being held by her mother, legs raised and screaming in pain as a woman leaned over her genitals, made me physically ill.

At that time there were several media reports of girls apparently being subjected to FGM in Australia, one in Western Australia and two in New South Wales. In two of these cases girls were allegedly taken to Indonesia for FGM. In the third the mutilation was done in NSW.

My new knowledge of the risks facing little girls in Australia burned in me. I had to do something!! I had never before felt such an urgency to act. Girls were possibly being mutilated right then in Australia!

I agree with the French term FGM as 'Female *Sexual* Mutilation'. That is exactly what FGM is aiming to do. I am outraged that some women are denied the human right to experience sexual pleasure.

I even however encountered nuanced arguments in Australia actually in support of FGM. I also needed to develop responses to questions about the legitimacy of my involvement as a white woman not from an FGM affected community.

The activities of No FGM Australia commenced with an online campaign including setting up a website with the help of Hilary Burrage, as well as a Facebook and Twitter page.

Twitter was a fantastic way to connect with others who were also fighting FGM, and I became an avid follower of the #FGM hashtags. Through Twitter hashtags such as

#FGM I began to connect with other international activists, particularly Hilary Burrage (UK), and then Tobe Levin (an American citizen living in Europe and Linda Weil-Curiel (France), the late Efua Dorkenoo (UK, through Equality Now), Ann-Marie Wilson, Ifrah Ahmed (Somalia/Ireland) and many others. I wanted to learn about FGM and how best to tackle it globally.

In terms of my understanding of FGM in Australia, my initial aim was to establish statistics on how much of a problem this really was.

One of the most supportive mentors I came across was Vivienne Strong, the manager for many years of the *NSW Education Program on FGM*. It is still one of the few in Australia which very clearly states on their website that FGM is child abuse and that if a girl is in danger the police should be called.

Around this time also Health Minister Tanya Plibersek and Prime Minister Julia Gillard were angry and outspoken about FGM, and they organised an 'FGM Summit', where my now-fellow No FGM Australia founder, Khadija Gbla, first spoke out about her experience as a survivor of FGM.

I contacted Khadija on LinkedIn, and we talked for hours. I realised it was essential that Khadija be the leading voice to speak against FGM, and we discussed setting up No FGM Australia as a formal organisation. Then we were also contacted by a Sydney businesswoman, Sybil Williams, who had lived in Africa, where her father had educated young men against FGM. The three of us together are the directors of the not-for-profit organisation, No FGM Australia.

In Australia, FGM was predominantly framed as a women's health issue, and there seemed to be a silence around the suggestion that FGM happens here. I was fortunate however to find friends internationally who were promoting the patriarchal underpinnings of FGM, that FGM is essentially a means to control women through reducing their sexuality. I was honoured to be part of a collaboration with the *Feminist Statement on FGM* (**www.statementonfgm.com**, 2013).

One problem when tackling FGM in Australia is that, unlike the UK, whilst the Australian Federal Police are responsible for acting if a girl is taken out of the country for FGM, when it comes to issues around child protection, health, education and police, each of these departments operates at a state, not a federal, level. There are eight separate governments dealing with FGM in eight different ways, all with different policies, systems and curricula, which need to be understood in order to protect girls from FGM.

But at least as campaigners we had three states covered. Khadija Gbla is based in South Australia, Sybil Williams in NSW and I myself in Victoria. We began to hold public awareness events, including in 2013 a screening of the powerful documentary made by Equality Now, *Africa Rising* when, along with our partners for the event, The Sydney Feminists, we secured speakers from African Women Australia, the NSW Education

Program on FGM, and No FGM Australia.

Soon we were joined by other volunteers in Brisbane, South Australia, NSW and Victoria.

No FGM Australia has now become legally incorporated as a company, with established aims and values and growing recognition as an organisation which aims to protect girls from FGM and empower survivors. We want *No FGM Australia* to become a sustainable company and we are seeking ways to maintain financial stability, which will enable us to fulfil our mission.

Khadija Gbla, now Executive Director of No FGM Australia, has been tireless, speaking out wherever people want to hear the vital voices of survivors campaigning against FGM.

In the past some Australians feared that involvement with the media might result in racism or the stigmatisation of those who come from a community affected by FGM, but we have found they consistently report incredibly sensitively on the subject, respecting Khadija's experiences and not sensationalising in any way. We see the media as an incredibly powerful tool for educating people about FGM. I have met any number of passionate young journalists who want to do their bit to stop FGM.

When speaking out against a culturally ingrained practice, survivors like Khadija do however risk massive backlash from their communities. It is considered taboo to talk about such a deeply personal topic, and yet it is only through strong survivor voices speaking out that people will come to listen and understand what a serious violation of human rights FGM really is.

One really positive aspect of my work as a campaigner against FGM is that I have met some wonderful people, such as Khadija Gbla, Hibo Wardere, Lucy Mashua and F.A. Cole, Ifrah Ahmed and Jeanette Sackey, whose story is told powerfully by Russell Traughber in *Driving the Birds*. It is critical that survivors of FGM such as Khadija, Lucy, Ifrah, Francess, Jeanette and Hibo are heard.

Beyond Australia, I have also been deeply involved via social media with grassroots NoFGM campaigns in Africa. One of these is the wonderful Pastoralist Child Foundation founded by Samuel Leadismo and Sayydah Garrett. In addition I've developed a strong bond with Sr Ephigenia Galachi, a Loreto nun who has striven for 15 years to educate the Maasai in her native Kenya about the harms of FGM and I also support the Lenkai Christian School (see Jackline) in Kenya.

We have a reasonably low rate of 15 per cent male infant circumcision in Australia, but I believe firmly that male infant circumcision is also child abuse and should not be legal and I am particularly distressed by the circumcisions on older boys in places such as the Philippines and parts of Africa. I do not, however, equate male circumcision with female genital mutilation. FGM is almost always in order to subjugate the woman and stop her from experiencing sexual pleasure.

Issues such as genital cosmetic surgery or piercing seem to me a distraction. The core issues are consent and purpose. Genital piercings and FGCS do not usually involve removal of the clitoris and do not result in destruction of sexual pleasure.

Recto-vaginal fistula is a different matter. Some organisations doing great work with women with fistula still deny the link between prolonged and obstructed labour (which results in obstetric fistula) and FGM. I want to see more research on recto-vaginal fistula and the extent to which FGM is a factor in this condition.

Currently we have little hard data on FGM in Australia but we have estimated conservatively that there are 1,100 girls per year born in Australia in circumstances placing them in extreme danger of undergoing FGM. We translated this to suggest that three girls a day are subjected to FGM.

Education through the law is as important as education in schools and we also need safeguarding strategies. I believe, like Waris Dirie, that the only way to properly protect girls is via regular medical checks, including the genitals. Then parents will then know for sure they will be caught, if they subject their daughter to FGM.

In 2014 No FGM Australia was recognised by the Australian Human Rights Commission for our work in Australia protecting girls and empowering survivors of FGM. This is an enormous thrill for all of us, and very affirming recognition that the Australian Human Rights Commission is also aware that FGM is a human rights issue facing Australian girls.

FGM is everyone's problem. We must not 'let' families decide whether they are going to mutilate their girls. All girls deserve to be safe. It's about the little girls, not their 'culture' or skin colour. I don't care if they are blue or green, they deserve to be protected. Abuse is abuse. Human rights are human rights.

FGM has got to stop.

***

Sybil Williams, an Australian business person, was born in Barbados. Her father worked for UNICEF, so she then lived in Nigeria, Burma, Nepal, Egypt, Lebanon, Bahrain and Wales before arriving in Australia in 1988 at the age of 15. Sybil recently joined Paula Ferrari and Khadija Gbla as a director of No FGM Australia.

***

My father worked for UNICEF when I was growing up, hence my multiple countries of residence as a child. Before that, however, one of his first jobs in his early twenties was as a science teacher in the Sudan. He rose to be a school inspector and would often be asked to take classes. One such class was teaching human reproduction, to 14-year-old boys.

Years later, whilst working for UNICEF (I was now in my early teens), my father took a three-month consultancy back in the Sudan. After finishing a day's workshop with a governmental body, one of the participants approached him.

'Do you remember me, Dr Williams?' the man asked. 'You, Dr Williams, have been the greatest source of trouble in my marriage.

'You gave a session on human reproduction to my class and during that class you banged your fist on the table and said, *'You are not a man if you allow your daughters to be cut! You are not a man!'*

'And, Dr Williams, my wife, my sister, my mother, my mother-in-law, my aunties and all my female relatives have not stopped giving me hell for it. But I wanted to tell you, my daughters are not cut, and neither are the daughters of anyone else in that room.'

That story made a huge impression on me. That's how I learnt about female genital mutilation.

Much later, I joined No FGM Australia when I learned – from what I can only consider now to be an incredibly naïve point of view – that FGM was occurring in Australia. I knew about FGM as a practice, but for some reason this additional information gave me the impetus to *do* something about it.

Now I'm a Director of No FGM Australia, with Paula Ferrari and our spokesperson, survivor Khadija Gbla. We work to protect young girls from the practice, and to support survivors. We have commissioned a report to estimate the prevalence of FGM within Australia and how many girls might be at risk.

I find FGM incredibly confronting and it makes me by turns very angry, very frustrated and very sad. At times, I have to dissuade myself from reading and learning more about it. I can find it overwhelming. I'm also keenly aware however that no matter how difficult I find thinking about FGM, I didn't have to go through it. I'm one of the lucky ones.

Nor do I kid myself that I am going to make much difference working within affected communities. As a white, middle class woman, that is probably not going to be where I will move the dial the most.

My aim is to bang the drum and get government not just to pay lip service, but to engage fully with the issue.

There is so much that could be done with a co-ordinated, cross-ministerial, federal and state government approach – but currently there's not a lot of political capital in it.

FGM is child abuse, sexual abuse, violence against women and a human rights issue. Protecting young girls and supporting survivors of this brutal crime is a role for everyone in a modern society.

Nonetheless, I also believe that practising communities themselves play an incredibly important role and these communities themselves know what is needed for those programmes. The anti-FGM programmes run in communities should be well funded by the government.

Cultural practices can change. One parallel I draw is to the Chinese practice of foot binding, which was also practiced for centuries. It was legislated against and it stopped.

The big difference is, of course, that it's much easier to see a bound foot than a cut clitoris – which makes the job that much more important. Teachers and doctors and nurses and social workers and the police and customs workers in Australia should all receive mandatory reporting training on how to recognise the danger signs of FGM, specifically, prior to the event, and on how to proceed if a girl has already been cut.

I would also like to see more (funded) work on replacing FGM with a ceremony which would be just as meaningful in order to celebrate a young woman's childhood / puberty / other milestone. I understand that this has been occurring in some communities in Africa, but I don't know if there has been much work within the diaspora on creating this alternative rite of passage.

People must understand that FGM is not solely a religious problem (although it's more common in some religions than others). It's a centuries-old practice with roots in some archaic notion of 'keeping women pure' by controlling their sexual feelings.

FGM is an Australian issue. I don't care how newly Australian the women are and neither should anyone else. It's not enough to announce new laws or introduce increased maximum sentencing.

If police don't understand what they're doing, if nurses and doctors don't ask or examine patients, and don't know what to do if they do find FGM, if teachers and social workers don't know the danger signs, or know what to do if they spot them and if customs personnel don't know where the legal lines are, there's a way to go. This needs a top down review and consistent policies across the board. That takes commitment and funding.

I want to get to the point where no one has to ask what FGM is, where it's accepted that FGM is a problem everyone should care about. We must move past anyone justifying FGM as a cultural practice and therefore, somehow, OK. What – like witch burnings?

Concern about condemning FGM is not somehow a racist position. In fact it's the opposite. If you would be outraged at the thought of your white daughter being mutilated in that – or any – way, why is it not racist to think it's OK for a child of African descent?

I want FGM to be something that people talk about and debate over the dinner table. I want it brought out of the 'women's issues' closet and into the sunlight of universal condemnation.

These things are all possible with education. The more people talk about the issue, the more widely it is known, the more likely the government is to prioritise funds for programmes to protect young girls and support their mothers.

Please talk about FGM to everyone, find a way to support activists, write letters and sign petitions. Make sure your government knows that this is an issue that matters.

....

Ms L was born in Australia and has first-hand experience of domestic violence. She currently works as a government lawyer. Her awareness of female genital mutilation was sharpened when she met Khadija Gbla at a No FGM Australia event, and she now volunteers with them when she can.

**

I am a lawyer working with an Australian government agency. I've been vaguely aware of female genital mutilation for many years, but the reality of it only struck me forcefully when I heard Khadija Gbla at a conference where she was a guest speaker.

Since that time I have become involved with Khadija's organisation, No FGM Australia, and I have given her what support I can (within the constraints of my job) in her current interactions with government agencies.

Things like FGM can only survive in the shadows. Awareness of this practice, and of how widespread and abhorrent it is, is key to its eradication. I personally find it offensive as we live in a society that does not value or respect female sexuality. FGM is child abuse pure and simple, a form of control over women.

Male privilege and patriarchy contribute to this practice but what I find so offensive is that women do this to other women! I appreciate that they are also usually victims themselves of course so the cycle of abuse continues and is intergenerational, making it very difficult to eradicate.

Decision makers must come to realise that FGM is not 'circumcision'. FGM is akin to lopping off the top third of a man's penis – if you are not OK with that, then you cannot be OK with FGM and still call yourself a civilised society.

The recent pronouncement by Sharia law advocates that only whores need a clitoris is so offensive I can barely find the words to respond.

Male circumcision is a totally different issue, for totally different reasons. But that said, I have concerns about both male and female 'circumcision'. Neither of my sons is circumcised. I had a partner in my twenties who was deeply emotionally scarred by the process. He has had been somewhat 'botched'.

People just don't understand what FGM entails. It is so difficult to discuss, that it becomes hidden in the shadows like domestic violence (DV) was years ago. I have myself come out of an abusive marriage. I am a DV survivor. My abuse was psychological and emotional in nature but in some ways that was more difficult to deal with as it took a long time to name and address the abuse for what it was.

Other issues such as female genital cosmetic surgery should be addressed separately. I think the pornification of women is to blame for this and I find such surgery abhorrent.

Women need to love themselves first and foremost. As with anything though we need to engage with men in an appropriate manner, though HeForShe and so on, to ensure these 'surgeries' are eradicated.

Most importantly, it's essential to raise awareness of FGM and take action to prosecute the people involved – no excuses - until it stops! It is not about being sensitive to cultural practices. That is a bullshit copout in my eyes.

This is child abuse and torture, it kills thousands of children a year. It's a form of genocide.

....

We have seen in this chapter, relating the development of the #EndFGM movement in Australia, how people are now grappling with the stark reality of FGM in one part of the western world. You can read more about the news and growing impact of the Australian campaign on the Female Mutilation Worldwide website. We now 'travel' to the USA and Canada, where campaigns to stop FGM, both domestically and in traditionally practising nations, are also stepping up.

In both Australia and North America, however, there remain people who insist that the eradication of FGM is disrespectful of centuries-long customs and that eradication should not therefore be enforced. This position continues to present challenges for campaigners, but their story overall is of significant accomplishments.

CHAPTER 7:

North America

There are probably around half a million women and girls who have experienced, or are at high risk of, FGM in the United States – the accurate figure is not known, but President Obama has recently confirmed that research will be carried out to ascertain a more precise figure.

Most of the contributors to this Chapter are United States Americans, some indigenous and some from very different origins; a few are Canadian. In 1994 Canada was the first country to recognise FGM as a form of persecution and the USA followed suit in 1996. FGM was made explicitly illegal in the USA in 1997, although not every state has explicitly done so even now. It is a conundrum that, despite the historic mix of peoples, there seems to be less acknowledgement of, or intelligence about, female genital mutilation in the USA than in, say, Britain. These narratives may suggest to readers a few of the reasons why that this is so.

THE SURVIVORS

We have already met F.A. Cole and Karima Amin, and now we hear from Lucy Mashua Sharp. All of them underwent female genital mutilation as children, in Sierra Leone and Yemen and Kenya respectively. They now all reside in the United States.

Lucy Mashua Sharp has been active in campaigns against FGM for many years, seeking the support of senators (including the then-new Senator Barack Obama) and other civic leaders across the political spectrum.

Lucy Mashua Sharp

We have over 280,000, perhaps twice that many, American girls (immigrants and their children) at risk of FGM. This is the highest number compared to other Western countries, yet there is less progress here because of racism.

I live in the United States now, but I come from the Rift Valley province, Kajiado South constituency of Kenya, where I was the first-born of six siblings, five sisters and one brother.

My environment when growing up was the beautiful jungles under the slopes of Mount Kilimanjaro. Every morning you wake up to this beautiful sight, where wild

100

animals and domestic animals run freely and the people cohabit with them. The sad thing is I feel safer with animals than with humans because, unlike the animals, the women and girls are not free. They are imprisoned in an unseen cage.

My childhood was robbed. I have selective amnesia and there are things I can't revisit because I am a survivor of female genital mutilation, which I underwent at the age of nine with a group of other Maasai girls. It was as painful as hell and I blanked out. Even now, my health is not good. I am frequently unwell with conditions related to FGM.

I don't think there is total healing. It is not even physical healing if your wounds heal but the scars remain open. That is why I get so angry when some political correctness zealots call it 'cutting' and 'circumcision'; I take that as an insult!

I only excuse FGM survivors, because I have no right to dictate to them how they should feel. Everyone else, I call them out: women don't have foreskins to be circumcised and also 'cutting' implies an accident, like the way you can 'accidentally' cut your finger. *Mutilation* however is intentional harm and / or pre-meditated murder, in this case to please a man.

Don't address me as a 'victim' I am now a 'survivor'. 'Victims' are the helpless girls and women being mutilated now, and those who bleed to death due to FGM.

Everyday more than eight thousand women and girls are mutilated in Africa alone. That is over three million annually. The World Health Organisation (WHO) must update their misleading global statistics, from the 140 million women and girls globally affected, an estimate that has not changed for the last three decades.

Then, still in Africa, there is breast ironing, where a hot iron is used to flatten women's breasts to stop them looking too female and sexual. There is teeth uprooting from the lower jaw where they take two middle teeth with pliers or a good manly fist blow so that a woman's smile cannot be too sexy. There is body marking and patterns with a red hot iron or knife to barbecue a woman's facial skin because having clear beautiful skin is too sexual, and women are sexual objects not sexual beings. There is the shaving of women's hair until bald, because hair is too sexual for women.

And in the Western developed world too, women are not valued. There is forced prostitution, brothels and massage parlours where women are pimped by men who take all of their money. Women are routinely discriminated against in jobs and hiring. The list goes on.

The majority of NGOs, often led by Westerners, who take their anti-FGM campaigns to Africa have done more harm than good. Some are very politically correct. Our people need to be told that what they are doing is against human rights. When dealing with Africans you don't beat around the bush.

Some of the NGOs spread propaganda and under-report the incidence of FGM. They spread false success to keep the funds from the USA / West coming. I have nothing good to say about them because they profit from pain.

Nor is spreading the anti-FGM message through the arts always going to work. East African artists are very different from West Africans because the majority of East African artists are religious singers and are quite conservative, whilst to the West the majority are secular musicians and more bold.

Standing against a tradition or ritual is still considered a taboo in my homeland community. You will make more enemies than friends. That's why I fled my homeland and went to safety in the USA. I had to leave my two very young children with their grandmother, and it was four long years before arrangements could be made for then to travel to the States to join me; but now we are a family again and they have a baby brother too.

When I first came to the USA I had so much hope for my cause and living the dream, which many Americans take for granted. Sometimes it feels that all they do is whine and complain of stupid petty stuff. So I arrived here (the USA) in 2006 and immediately I began a mission for my homeland. That is how I became 'Global Ambassador Against FGM'.

Unless the campaign is spearheaded by whites you get no support at all; racism in human rights is just pathetic. So I decided to do my own thing and not to wait for anybody, because girls and women continue to suffer and die every day. Time waits for no one.

I started a radio show where I only talk about FGM, in English and Kiswahili. It reaches immigrants and Africans globally. I blog about FGM too; and that is how I mediate many different concerns.

I was shocked that many people here didn't know about FGM and still don't. Even many immigrants feel no need to talk about FGM; only a handful care.

I am not sure whether this ignorance is because they are ignorant, or whether it's because we are talking about things that don't happen to them personally, so they couldn't care less. Maybe it's the shock, as they can't believe this atrocity still happens. Maybe they are racists, because even after many of them know they don't give a toss. Or maybe it's because we are talking about vaginas.

Gynaecologists should be very gentle and thoughtful when dealing with survivors, because we re-live FGM when our legs are apart and it feels as though they are chained onto the examination table.

I remember my first gynaecology visit. The doctor was a male and when he was about to insert a penis-shaped sonogram instrument into my vagina he whispered, 'Oh my god, I don't know what I am dealing with here'. He'd told me nothing about what he was going to do or what the hell a sonogram was. I was never prepared psychologically at all., so my defence mechanism kicked in and I jumped like a ninja from the table, pushed the doctor with my foot and ran out of the room with the hospital gown still open from behind, giving people in the corridor and the waiting room a show.

I am an expert witness in immigration courts for FGM and human rights in general. Some immigration officers, judges and police officers are very insensitive, and the main reason is they think FGM really doesn't happen and they cannot fathom it or process the details they hear.

I salute Europe, particularly the UK, for the excellent work they are all doing. Here in the US they are still lazy and unwilling. The UK has led for example in working with survivors and letting their voices lead the way. But universal discrimination remains when it comes to funding.

Thank you to all who provide repairs of fistula, hernia, vagina keloids, fibroids, cysts and scar tissues. You are all lifesavers.

The fight against FGM should be centre stage. Push it to every media wave, write and call, talk about it, get tougher laws and prosecute, jail the mutilators, print flyers and more.

FGM should be talked about every single day until it's history. One excellent example of this dialogue was the meeting of FGM activists and academics, Contestations around FGM: Activism and the Academy, organised by Dr Tobe Levin at Oxford University for International Women's Day, on 7th March 2015.

I am so happy to see a global spotlight to expose FGM atrocities. God bless the women of this world and the gender sensitive men.

....

OTHER NORTH AMERICAN CAMPAIGNERS

Amongst the vigorous campaigners against female genital mutilation in the United States are also a number who are not themselves victims or survivors of the practice. Taina Bien-Aimé, who holds a doctorate in law, is an American citizen of Haitian descent. Currently Executive Director of the *Coalition Against Trafficking in Women* (CATW) in New York, Taina was also a founding board member and later Executive Director of Equality Now. She refers here to the new generation of activists such as Jaha Dukureh (USA) and Leyla Hussein (UK).

Like Taina Bien Aimé, in addition to campaigning against FGM Karen Lambie is deeply concerned about human trafficking. Karen lives in Georgia, USA and has qualifications in Educational Psychology. She is a retired teacher with three decades of experience and is now a foster parent.

Angela Peabody was born in Liberia, where she remained until as an adult a violent coup d'état forced her and her family to flee. She is Founder-President of the US-based non-profit organisation Global Woman P.E.A.C.E. Foundation, and, as A.M. Peabody, has written two award-winning novels, *Exiled: In the Bowels of American Society* (2004) and *When the Games Froze* (2014).

Barbara Mhangami-Ruwende, also now a writer, was born in Zimbabwe and studied medical biochemistry in Britain before she arrived in the USA in 1997 for post-graduate research in epidemiology and public health. Barbara founded the Africa Research Foundation for the Safety of Women (AFRSW). She reminds us that FGM takes many forms. The less usual ones, such as labia elongation, are classified as 'Type 4'.

Taine Bien-Aimé

My maternal grandmother was a suffragist. She instilled in my mother, who then transmitted to her daughters a strong sense of independence and a quest for justice and equality.

A first generation American, I learned early that education was key in one's life journey toward fulfilment and purpose. At ten years old, I moved to Geneva, Switzerland, where I lived and studied until 24 years of age. Upon my return back to New York and a few years working for an international organisation that focussed on development across African nations, I enrolled in law school after which I joined a Wall Street law firm.

For the past two decades I have had the privilege to work with other passionate advocates for the rights of women and girls, including the late and beloved Efua Dorkenoo. It was in New York in 1992 that I met and joined with the co-founder of Equality Now, Jessica Neuwirth, who with two other attorneys shared the vision to address all forms of violence and discrimination against women and girls as human rights violations. 22 years later, my passion remains, with great hope for a safer world for women and girls worldwide and my two beloved sons.

Today, as Executive Director of the Coalition Against Trafficking in Women (CATW), I continue my work to ensure equality for all. CATW is the first and oldest international non-governmental organisation dedicated to ending trafficking in women and girls and related forms of commercial sexual exploitation as practices of gender-based violence.

My work on ending FGM continues with our support for Jaha Dukureh, an outstanding young human rights leader and survivor of FGM who formed the organisation Safe Hands for Girls.

My enduring wish is to eradicate female genital mutilation everywhere. Without a doubt, the UK is ahead of the USA in this struggle; some ground-breaking work is being undertaken there.

I disagree however with the suggestion by some British activists that we cannot stop FGM in Western countries until it has been eradicated in places where it is traditionally practised. As Eleanor Roosevelt once said, 'Human rights begins at home,' so it is our responsibility to end human rights violations, including FGM, wherever we live.

Recent work in the UK by the Health and Social Care Information Centre (HSCIC) to elucidate the incidence of FGM, in England at least, needs to be replicated in the USA and elsewhere. My young friend Jaha Dukureh's e-petition requesting such a move, and President Obama's response to develop a comprehensive strategic plan to end the practice in the US, are promising efforts.

Legally, in the USA and in many countries, the practice of FGM on minors is child abuse and all violence against women and girls is also a crime. Detecting these crimes and bringing the perpetrators to justice however is not easy, nor is there clarity about how to deal with those who genitally mutilate girls.

US federal law provides some protection for children (including girls at risk of FGM, via the *Girls' Protection Act*, which expressly forbids anyone from taking a child abroad for FGM), but only 22 states have specific legislation against FGM and to date, there are no established preventive measures, including education about the harms of FGM.

FGM is a 5,000-year-old harmful cultural practice that precedes the Judeo-Christian and Muslim religions and traditions. Even when the diaspora from FGM-practicing communities know about laws prohibiting FGM, the cultural fears and superstitions that maintain the practice of FGM make it difficult to combat it.

Further, survivors of FGM often do not make the connections between FGM and the myriad physical, physiological and psychological ailments they endure as a direct result of the harmful practice. Investing in outreach and education about women's health, including sexual and reproductive health, is key in these communities.

The term 'women's rights are human rights' was only coined in 1993 at the United Nations World Conference on Human Rights in Vienna. We have made considerable strides in the twenty or so years since then. The medical community now recognises better the impact of FGM and other harmful practices against girls and women, and, with the growth of social media, young anti-FGM activists such as Leyla Hussain and Jaha Dukureh are far more visible than their foremothers in the struggle. Although resistance is a measure of a success, it remains fierce in our collective efforts to end FGM.

The worldwide web is making a massive difference to what together we can all achieve, tying grassroots efforts to policymakers to the public consciousness about FGM. There is hope.

We need strong government responses to FGM and other gender-based harmful practices. The movement also desperately needs financial support, in particular for activists at the grassroots level. There is a way to go.

***

Karen Lambie

Even before I left work, I knew I wanted to use my retirement to speak against child abuse issues and violations of human rights.

I foster children and am required to take a certain number of training hours every year to maintain my status as a foster parent for the state of Georgia. During one of our training sessions, the woman conducting the session told us about a case in Georgia in which an infant became a victim of female genital mutilation while in foster care.

The FGM was done by one of this child's older sisters with a heated coat hanger, which was used to burn off the infant's clitoris. When the sister was asked why she had mutilated her infant sister, she said if they ever returned to Somalia, she wanted to make sure her sister was marriageable. I sat listening to this tale in total disbelief, my mouth open with tears flowing down my face.

Many, many years ago I read an insert about FGM in a college textbook so I had heard of it before, but had I been asked about it, I would have said I'm sure it isn't even practiced anymore. After my course that day I felt compelled to get more information. This report was of a case that had happened right here in my own state.

While doing research on the subject of FGM, I came across an online community called A Safe World for Women, which was founded by Chris Crowstaff. One of the issues addressed by Safe World was female genital mutilation.

You can imagine my absolute shock when I found out how prevalent it still is in certain parts of the world. That was all it took. I needed to do something about it. I needed to stand up for my global sisters.

As I began reading articles, I discovered that, because of their cultural heritage, it is estimated that there are some 250,000 girls or more, right here in the United States, at risk of this barbaric procedure. I could not believe what I was reading. I also discovered that there are thousands of girls at risk who live in the UK and Australia.

I was not (and still am not) part of an organisation with the specific objective of fighting FGM. I am an individual, but I could not sit back and do nothing.

I learned as much as I could and put together a presentation and handouts about FGM. I had business-type cards made and started passing them out to friends. I was asked to speak to a few women's organisations and to host booths at several health fairs in Savannah, Georgia.

When I speak or host a booth, I give out a lot of information on FGM, including websites where people can go to learn more. I have books written on the subject. I put them on display as well.

Many, many people that I have spoken to have no idea what I'm talking about. When I explain FGM, they stare at me with wide eyes and gapping mouths. They cannot believe what they are hearing.

Every once in a while, I will meet someone who not only knows about it, but knows someone who has undergone the procedure and knows how horrible it is.

Two things come up over and over again when talking about FGM: economics and ignorance. In regard to economics, we need to eradicate poverty among women. For ignorance, we need to educate leaders and citizens of cultures in which it is still practised.

I know this is much easier said than done. Economics, poverty and the lack of education are very closely tied. In many ways, FGM is tied very closely to economic factors. We absolutely need to eradicate poverty among women.

In my research, I have learned that a main reason for continuing FGM is because the 'cutters', who are mostly women, get paid. This is their livelihood. Also, without the 'cut' women cannot marry, and will become an economic burden.

I was also very shocked to learn about the many myths concerning the female genitalia, such as that, if not cut off, the clitoris will continue to grow down to the woman's knees. This is where education definitely needs to play a part. People in these cultures also need to learn that many of the complications women suffer after the procedure are *because* of the procedure.

Although I am not a victim of FGM myself, I have very strong feelings about it. It's one of the most barbaric practices I have ever heard of. In my opinion it is one of the most extreme and severe violations of human rights on the planet.

I will continue to raise awareness, keep signing petitions and encourage others to do the same. In addition to campaigning against female genital mutilation I am an Ambassador of Hope To End Human Trafficking (Shared Hope International). There is nothing I want more than to see FGM and human trafficking come to an end.

***

Angela Peabody

Angela Peabody is an award-winning novelist who was born in Liberia, where she remained until as an adult a violent coup d'état forced her and her family to flee. She has lived in the United States for the past 34 years.

I have lived in the United States for the past 34 years. I am Founder-Director of the Global Woman P.E.A.C.E. Foundation, which now organises the annual #EndFGM Walk-A-Thon in Washington. DC.

As a child living in Liberia, my sisters and I were fortunate that our parents did not believe in female genital mutilation, so we were spared; but I now know so many survivors to whom I feel close.

I didn't then understand what it was, but I first became aware of FGM more than 50 years ago, in my homeland when I was eight. A playmate disappeared and my friends and I didn't know what had happened to her. Two years later, she reappeared but she was not the same pleasant and happy girl. I will never forget the sadness in her eyes.

There were rumours that my little friend had been taken to the 'Grebo Bush' and her private parts had been cut off, cooked and given to her to eat, but she never spoke about it to us. I was curious about the rumours but too afraid to ask anyone, for fear that I too would be abducted and taken to the Grebo Bush. I recall seeing girls walking around wearing only G-strings and topless, with their entire bodies covered with white chalk.

Later I learned that the Grebo Bush is where members of the Sande Society take girls to undergo female genital mutilation in preparation for womanhood, but my playmate eventually passed away without marriage and children. She never disclosed what had happened to her in the Grebo Bush. She never admitted even being there. The Sande Society in Liberia is a deeply rooted cultural secret society. They instil in the girls never to tell anyone what happened to them, otherwise they will die.

Then I forgot about the Grebo Bush and the fear until, many years later after immigrating to the US, I read about a high fashion model from Somalia who had survived something called female genital mutilation, or 'female circumcision'. This FGM survivor made a heroic escape from her Somalian village, fleeing her country. Finally I realised what had really happened to my playmate many years before.

My growing realisation of the hurt, which her genital mutilation caused to my little friend in Liberia drove me to enquire further and to campaign against FGM. With an education and previous professional experience in broadcast journalism, I decided in April 2014 to take early retirement to work full-time with our organisation, Global Woman P.E.A.C.E. Foundation.

In 2014 I authored a novel, *When the Games Froze*, about FGM. Afterwards, at a focus group meeting held by our organisation, several young women approached me and disclosed for the first time that they had been mutilated when they were between the ages of seven and nine. They felt my book had inspired them to share their stories.

My and I put on the first '*Walk to End FGM*' in the US on 8 November, 2014. We are preparing to put on the second on 31 October, 2015. This will become an annual event to help raise awareness about FGM.

Global Woman P.E.A.C.E. Foundation has also partnered with the organization *Clitoraid*, to help raise funds to sponsor restorative surgery for FGM survivors. The cost for each person is $1700 in the US and $300 in Africa. We are committed to assisting these young women to get through the physical scars, as well as the psychological scars they tend to live with for the rest of their lives.

In June 2015 we will open the *Global Woman Center* in Washington, D.C., where women and girls can find refuge, counselling, obstetric and gynaecological referrals, and restorative surgery. We will invite immigrant mothers to visit the Center and provide information on the dangers of FGM without antagonizing them.

Tragically, FGM in the USA is not becoming less common at all. The majority of Americans rely on the media to learn about the things going on around them, and the

US media could really help if they wanted to. So far, major media coverage has not materialized at all.

The US Department of Education could also help a great deal if they allowed us to teach FGM in the schools. Teachers, school counsellors and local police departments should be educated on FGM and that will help prevent it from occurring.

We need to reach schools, university campuses, the faith-based community, the major media market in the US and the sports arenas (athletes have a lot of influence). Perhaps people see FGM as an African problem or an Asian or Middle Eastern problem, but I disagree. It is now an American problem, a European problem and a problem of the world.

I want mainstream society to become actively involved in stopping FGM, and the other two harmful traditional practices (HTPs) of which I am aware, breast-ironing and child marriage. Child marriage is associated with FGM, and breast-ironing is done in an effort to prevent girls' breasts from growing. It is very prevalent in Cameroon and is held to protect girls' 'purity'.

I want global recognition that FGM is an atrocious and heinous act on innocent little girls.

Liberia, my country of birth, is the oldest African independent republic. It should have been the country to set an example by making the practice of FGM unlawful. Instead, politicians in that country support FGM, and as a result the practice has escalated in the last twenty years. Liberian leaders should work with the Sande Society to reach agreement to eliminate FGM from the Grebo Bush training which they regard as required for womanhood.

The United States is, however, my current country of residence, and whilst I applaud the current administration for starting the FGM conversation, there remains a great deal to be done.

People in the United States are not talking about FGM. They cannot even bring themselves to utter the words 'female genital mutilation'. FGM is very foreign to Americans.

I dream that schoolteachers and counsellors and police officers will be specifically trained to help protect at-risk girls in the USA. I want recognition that FGM is proper and valid grounds for asylum.

I want to see our *Washington Global Woman Center* really help survivors of FGM. We aim to establish a network of trained obstetricians and gynaecologists in the US who will make the FGM survivors comfortable during medical examinations, and when performing the restorative surgeries.

We also need to be aware of fistula. I support restorative surgeries for FGM related conditions because they give survivors relief from ongoing physical pain and help prevent infant and maternal mortalities.

Sometimes a comparison is made between FGM and male circumcision, but in my opinion male circumcision is different from FGM. There is a medical purpose for male circumcision. It is a matter of cleanliness because dirt and bacteria can accumulate under the foreskin if it remains in place. The alternative to male circumcision is to teach the boys how to clean under the foreskin from an early age.

There is however no medical reason to remove the clitoris and/or the labia. It is not a matter of cleanliness with the female genitalia. I think males try to compare male circumcision to FGM as a way to divert attention from FGM and lessen its magnitude.

I want to see a major movie made about FGM, and more literature. I appeal to everyone who is knowledgeable about FGM to begin the conversation with those who are not. If you sit next to someone on a flight or a train, a bus, in a restaurant, at the club, at church, ask her or him if they have ever heard of female genital mutilation. That will start the conversation, and you just might win over a new advocate or campaigner.

***

Barbara Mhangami-Ruwende

We are not angry enough about FGM. Why are we not shutting down governments, churches, media houses, with our primal screams for this atrocity to end?

The issue of FGM and violence against women is always in my consciousness. It is front and centre of all I do and talk about. It breaks my heart. Most times I am asking, *'Where is the outrage?'*

FGM is at the core of the destruction of the feminine and this to me is the greatest crime and threat to our humanity, the destruction of the feminine.

I was born and spent my childhood in Zimbabwe, where I first became aware of female genital mutilation as such when I was about fourteen 14 years old. By 'FGM' I mean 'cutting', which is different from the practice in several Southern African countries including Zimbabwe, whereby the labia minora are elongated by pulling with the fingers.

Labia elongation usually happens in girls aged about nine to thirteen, before the first period. It is a sort of initiation into womanhood, a preparation for marriage because long labia are supposed to be attractive to men and they mark the distinction between a woman and a girl. The older women are responsible for teaching girls how to do this and along with this teaching usually comes instruction on how to please a man sexually.

The actual process may not always be painful, but of course it is not right to force children to change their bodies, particularly if it is not medically indicated and of no benefit to them as individuals.

My direct involvement with female genital mutilation in the usual sense came when I lived in Europe and I spent a lot of time with people from Francophone West Africa.

A friend from Guinea talked about FGM as a positive thing that happened to her and recounted her experience of it. I could not conceive of what a mutilated vagina might look like and she offered to show me hers. I was totally changed from that day on. At 22, I knew that FGM was what I would devote my time and effort to speaking out against for the rest of my life.

I now live in the USA, where I am Founder of the Africa Research Foundation for the Safety of Women. Part of what we do is to look at creative approaches to ending FGM, particularly here in the United States among marginalised immigrant communities.

My research background as a scientist, and my cultural competency training, will be of great use in this project.

It is hard to measure FGM in the communities that I know of because they are largely closed communities. Many of the women and girls are non-English speaking and the issue of immigration status makes it very difficult to gain the trust of these communities enough to broach the subject of FGM. It took me nine years to gain the trust of the women from West Africa around the Detroit Metro Area.

Last year, on 8 November, 2015, we partnered with the Global Women P.E.A.C.E Foundation founded by an amazing Liberian woman, Angela Peabody, in the first ever walk against FGM in Washington DC. This event was to raise awareness of the issue of FGM in the United States and to highlight the girls who are at risk of 'vacation cutting'. I spoke at this event and, this year, plans are already underway for more collaborative work around identifying marginalised communities and ways to reach those at risk in these communities.

Counselling centres and training of medical and school personnel are also underway so that we take a systematic multi-pronged approach to the issue, rather than shooting in the dark and wasting precious time and resources.

That FGM should be condemned is indisputable. It is a gross violation of women and children's rights and it is a criminal offence. The manner in which this is done must, however, be sensitive to the negative consequences that direct attacks on groups or particular religions can bring. The potential for stigmatisation of those who have had it done or those who do it has to be monitored and addressed.

One huge consequence is that if stigmatisation occurs the practice will simply go underground and children will be cut as babies. Another consequence particularly in the diaspora is that FGM will become a defining component of identity in communities away from the mainstream.

We need endorsement at the highest level of the right of women to remain intact. In Burkina Faso that endorsement was provided by the wife of the President. In the States, we have the pronouncements of Barack Obama, from the letter he wrote before his election as President of the USA to Lucy Mashua Sharp, through to his confirmation in office that the large-scale study demanded by Jaha Dukureh of the incidence of FGM in the States will be conducted.

But endorsement is not enough. Many nations have laws against FGM. Few have routinely enforced them, as the case of Egypt, where FGM has become largely medicalised, demonstrates well.

On the practical side legalistically, we need to see transnational collaboration. We know that girls are transported between nations for the mutilation, and that the diaspora has resulted in a significant increase in the numbers of children at risk in the USA. For some FGM has become a tragic marker of their heritage.

Those who harm their girls must be punished, but I want to see transformative justice, not retribution.

The solution to these challenges will be educating key influential members in these communities. These people, men and women, leaders and 'cutters' included, can then educate others in the community as well.

Readers of this book must help us by sharing information about FGM with their friends, families and co-workers. Everyone can look for ways to get involved in their own communities to raise awareness, and to offer support to survivors and those who are at risk for FGM, always taking the lead from the women and girls themselves, as to what needs to be done.

....

INTERNATIONAL CAMPAIGNERS

All three USA-based campaigners working to stop female genital mutilation in parts of Africa have partnered with men from or in the countries – Somalia and Kenya – concerned. Julie Barton became involved, alongside Ahmed Hassan who also lives in Minneapolis, in a non-profit organisation called Action for Women and Child Concern (AWCC), to stop FGM in the local Somali population in their US hometown, and amongst women and girls in Somalia.

Both Sayydah Garrett and Teri Gabrielsen found their lives changed after chance encounters whilst on safari in Kenya and, independently, both have founded organisations to prevent FGM and promote education. Sayydah, a Canadian, now resident in the USA, collaborates with Samuel Leadismo on the Pastoralist Child Foundation programme in the Samburu and Maasai tribal communities; and Teri, an American, is a qualified school teacher who created with a Kenyan male leader the charity Africa Schools of Kenya (ASK) in Maasailand, Kenya.

Ahmed and Samuel are both, with Sayydah and Teri, seeking to eradicate FGM, a major obstacle to girls remaining in school, via Alternative Rites of Passage (which are often referred to as ARPs).

Julie Barton

It was in Minnesota public library, in October 2012, that I heard Naomi Wolf speak about her new book, *Vagina: A New Biography*. 'If your goal is to break a woman psychologically, it is efficient to do violence to her vagina,' was her message, as she spoke about rape, sexual violence and FGM.

I couldn't stop thinking about that. I had just begun a Master of Liberal Studies programme at Metropolitan University. I did a lot of reading about FGM and searched for experts in the field. The first person I reached out to was Hilary Burrage.

My capstone project became a research paper on FGM and I graduated with my Masters (Liberal Studies) in May 2015. As I've reached the end of my programme, I realise I still need the tools to do what I hope to accomplish. I will begin a Master of Public Affairs program at the University of Minnesota Humphrey Institute in Fall 2015. I will then be able to take forward policy proposals about FGM.

I also joined Action for Women and Child Concern (AWCC), based in Somalia. AWCC's mission is to eradicate poverty, extreme hunger, illiteracy, inequalities and empowering women and children to reach their full potential. I agreed to partner with another Minnesotan, Ahmed Hassan, on condition that we make FGM education a priority.

Minneapolis, Minnesota, has the largest Somali diaspora outside of Somalia. My top priority is to educate our community that FGM is an issue. I am currently working with a group of Somali women who have shared their survivor stories with a reporter for the *Star Tribune* newspaper.

When I originally talked to the *Star Tribune* reporter about new Somali refugees coming to Minnesota, I was told that FGM is not a problem here. When I pressed her on it, she said that it is illegal. After hearing the Somali women speak about their experiences of FGM and pressures from family members to send their children back to Somalia to undergo FGM, she now recognises the realities of FGM and is trying to figure out the best way to present this issue.

Hibo Wardere, an FGM survivor from Somalia who is now based in Britain, also gave an interview for AWCC's newsletter *Innocent Voices*.

Right now, not many people feel FGM is a problem in Minnesota. The community, if they even know about it, believe that FGM only happens in Africa. They do not realise the refugees suffer from the effects FGM, but FGM can't be eradicated without it becoming an issue for the mainstream, along with being tackled within traditionally practising communities.

Nonetheless, Somali women who have been speaking to our local reporter feel very nervous about talking about FGM. I want to give them a voice, but they are afraid they will lose friends and become ostracised from their community for speaking out.

I am continually learning new things. I am looking forward to reading about other's successes and seeing if I can replicate these here and in Somalia.

***

Sayydah Garrett

The term 'female genital mutilation' wasn't used, but about 12 years ago I saw a documentary where a girl was undergoing FGM. My whole body shuddered. I just couldn't (and never will) believe my eyes – the horror!!

Some years later I took a vacation to see the savannah grasslands in Kenya, and there I met Samuel Leadismo, who works as a visitor guide. Samuel told me about the enduring problem of FGM in his tribal community, the Samburu, and asked me to help him change things.

I am Canadian but have lived in the USA for many years. When I returned to the USA, I founded a non-profit organisation, Pastoralist Child Foundation, to eradicate FGM and child marriage in the Samburu and Maasai tribal communities in Kenya, working with Samuel in his homeland.

Our organisation provides educational workshops for girls during school holidays to teach the harmful effects of FGM. Detailed explanations, pictures and plastic models of the female genital area are shown to demonstrate precisely the procedure.

We have visited local primary schools to talk to young girls about FGM and forced marriage. We provide educational workshops for women, to teach the short and long-term effects of FGM and to encourage them to reconsider the continued practice with their daughters. We also sponsor girls' education and currently have 5 girls receiving full scholarships to attend private and national secondary boarding schools.

Girls in Kenya often leave school, because they are married after FGM, or when their periods start. We fight early marriage and also provide practical support like sanitary napkins, so they can stay on. Then FGM rates will drop.

Our organisation partners with other local anti-FGM grassroots organisations with the same mission. On International Women's Day in 2014 we collaborated with Caritas Maralal (Catholic Diocese of Maralal, Samburu County, Kenya – see Lucy Espila) to talk to the audience about FGM.

Then, on February 6, 2015, the annual International Day of Zero Tolerance against FGM, our organisation sent a delegation of men, women, youths and elders to Maralal to join thousands of other like-minded individuals and organisations, to demonstrate our commitment to accelerating the abolishment of FGM.

We must educate Muslims who still believe FGM is part of their faith, when in fact it *isn't* a requirement in Islam. We need more Muslim clerics to state that FGM is unacceptable in Islam.

Girls are extremely marginalised in the highly patriarchal society in which they live. It's time for their voices to be heard. It's time for them to stand up against an act of violence that harms them physically, psychologically, and emotionally for the rest of their lives. By replacing FGM with safe Alternative Rites of Passage, which we call ARPs, the life outcomes of girls will greatly improve!

The traditional communities concerned do make it difficult to speak out. It has been historically taboo to talk about FGM. Elders are highly respected and what they say must be obeyed, without question.

Rape, domestic abuse/violence, assault, sexual abuse, molestation, and murder are acts of violence that all societies work to end. Why not the same for FGM, whether in Kenya, the USA or Canada? The victims are almost all children. We must ensure these children are properly protected.

Pastoralist Child Foundation looks forward to the day when FGM is completely eradicated. We know that realistically it will take several more years but, for every girl that is saved from FGM because of the collective work of so many individuals and organisations around the world working feverishly to eradicate it, it's worth it.

Whilst FGM rates are gradually declining, there are still six thousand girls a day being mutilated around the world, and millions more at risk. This must end!

We will continue our work to raise awareness about FGM in the United States and Canada, because some immigrants from Africa, the Middle East, the Sub-Continent and even Europe are practising FGM. They are also sending girls to their home countries to be mutilated during school holidays. There's a new term for it – 'vacation cutting'.

Organisations and individuals working to end FGM in the USA and Canada must keep the pressure on their respective governments to enforce the law. If perpetrators are caught, they must suffer the consequences, should they be found guilty in a court of law.

On behalf of Pastoralist Child Foundation, I would like to take this opportunity to thank Hilary Burrage for her continued campaign against FGM. I would also like to thank each and every individual and organisations (grass roots, community based organisations, NGOs, non-profits, etc.) working to eradicate this terrible vice called FGM.

The best thing to do in the communities in which we work, in rural Kenya, is to continue educating girls, women, boys, men and elders about the very harmful effects of FGM.

Education = Empowerment = Equality.

***

Teri Gabrielsen

It was in 2007, as an American tourist on safari in Kenya, that I first met James Ole Kamete, an elder of the Maasai Esiteti community. James was determined that both boys and girls who are living in Esiteti be educated – an unusual ambition because education was traditionally reserved for only boys.

And so began our partnership with Africa Schools of Kenya (ASK), a non-profit organisation which I, a qualified teacher, founded to deliver educational programmes and scholarships for the children of the Esiteti and Mbaringoi communities in Maasailand. ASK also works to eradicate female genital mutilation, a major obstacle to girls remaining in school, via Alternative Rites of Passage (ARPs).

The ARP curriculum was developed by ASK and the Esiteti village women elders, including the 15 'cutters' in the area. The ARP was piloted as a two-day programme in August, 2012. It is facilitated by a trained Maasai nurse and a college educated Maasai from outside the Esiteti area. These two professionals act as ARP facilitators leading discussions with 25 participants on various aspects of subjects concerning the female body. Every ARP since 2012 has followed the traditional *Emuratare* rituals, except FGM is no longer performed.

These group lessons and discussions include maturation changes in the female and male bodies, the myths and misperceptions of FGM as a rite of passage for a girl to become a women in the eyes of her community, how HIV/AIDS is sexually and otherwise transmitted, issues involving rape, the health risks of early pregnancy and early marriage, family planning options, the illegality of FGM in Kenyan law, physical violence, self-esteem issues and the importance of an education through secondary school and college. Similarly, parents learn about the health risks of FGM and the importance of their daughters' education.

FGM is now being replaced with education, and education is now the new coming of age for young women living in the Esiteti area.

Several of the ARP graduates have been selected to lead a peer-to-peer ARP training programme, so they can learn the necessary tools to duplicate the ARP model and expand the ARP programme throughout Maasailand. One of the students, Nelly, caught our attention years back, because she had convinced her mother and father she wanted to remain in school and not go through the traditional *Emuratare* involving FGM.

Nelly's family was ostracised by the Esitety community members for being different, but now things have changed and she and her parents are 'leaders' to the Esiteti community. Nelly will be trained to introduce the ARP model to other communities to the southern region of Kenya, reaching a projected 13,000 girls a year throughout Maasailand.

We want to stop FGM as soon as possible. We plan to implement Alternative Rites of Passage (ARPs) for a projected 13,000 girls a year throughout Maasailand. To achieve this goal we will require significant resourcing. We are currently seeking substantial grant funding to scale up ASK's ARP model, and one grant application with the Bill & Melinda Gates Foundation is pending.

Education, education, education is our plan. As these ARP graduates and young women counsel their peers throughout Maasailand, girls and women will have the tools to make their communities even more prosperous.

....

MEDIA AND THE ARTS

The 'stories' of people whose lives have been touched by female genital mutilation are compelling. For many FGM changes their experience permanently. Diane Walsh is a Canadian and an internationally accredited journalist, artist and painter. She often choses to support those who tell their stories through story-telling, narrative and the arts, as does Tobe Levin (next chapter), an American living in Germany who also works in the UK.

Diane, like Tobe, challenges directly the obdurate 'social relativism' which has developed, especially in many North American university campuses, on issues around FGM. They (and, indeed, the writer of this book) disagree profoundly with the social relativist, non-judgemental, approach adopted by some anthropologists and other academics and activists, which holds that every culture has its own culture and ethics, and social beliefs therefore have no absolute moral truth or validity. Tobe Levin calls this a-moral position '*Anthr/Apology*'. But FGM is not, Diane and Tobe both rightly insist, a matter about which it is ethically or morally acceptable to take a non-judgemental or detached position. As Cath Holland will also remind us, it is fundamentally unacceptable to sit on the fence when children's lives and futures are at stake.

Diane is an internationally accredited journalist and an artist, a painter.

Diane Walsh

I read *Gyn/Ecology: The Metaethics of Radical Feminism* by Mary Daly (Beacon Press, 1978) back in Montréal whilst I was completing my college studies. One of the chapters was on female genital mutilation.

My reaction was frozen in time. I was horrified that such a thing could be done to womankind and I vowed that one day I would do something about it. I was deeply disturbed by the chapter and especially by the fact that no one at that time in the

Western academy (i.e. within the wider 'classical liberal cannon' of literature and academic research) seemed to be talking openly about FGM in the way that Daly had courageously done.

Needless to say I later learned about all the backlash and the bizarre political wars then apparent in North American university radical feminism, including attitudes towards Betty Dobson who challenged the feminist writer and activist, Gloria Steinem.

The fact was, no second-wave liberal American feminists were willing back then to take on FGM. This was cultural relativism at its worst!

I am a global citizen of Irish, French Canadian and Scottish descent, with a mission to help stop FGM and also an artist. My art on FGM and other political themes has been exhibited in London UK, at the UN and in Geneva and Vancouver Island Canada.

As an international correspondent I split my time between Washington DC, Europe and Canada (where, except when the family travelled in Europe, I lived as a child). I now have a decade of experience as a watchdog journalist and archivist/researcher.

Focussing on Political Theory, Ethnography Studies/feminist methodologies and then Social Anthropology whilst a student in Canada, I drew particularly on the work of the highly regarded sociologist Dorothy Smith, whose method(s) of inquiry, including writings on Institutional Ethnography I plan to apply also to my further academic research around FGM.

It's taken decades but now finally FGM is at the forefront of academic thought, exemplified (you could say) by the 7 March, 2015 event at Oxford University, Contestations around FGM: Activism and the Academy which, as one excellent and positive example, pooled together extraordinary activists from around the world. Praxis is reborn!

In my own life, I have travelled to the United Nations in New York and Geneva (in both of which campuses I have media accreditation), Paris, France, Ireland, and of course the UK, chasing the issue. I have been active in the anti-FGM movement quite definitively since 2009 but really it's been a life-long endeavour to break the silence. I am active in the Global Alliance Against FGM (GA-FGM) and I contribute articles, art and raise awareness in a multitude of ways, social media, walks, talks, and outreach of every kind.

We must stop at nothing to stop FGM. Genocide on one woman is genocide on all women. We can't stand idle. This is the creed.

Much can be done to eradicate FGM in the Western countries. There must be a broad and holistic approach, both trans-disciplinary and inter-disciplinary. The UK has the start of a solid template but it must be in conjunction with the US and the United Nations in Geneva.

More awareness does seem to be helping. Arrests are gradually being made. I give particular credit to the UK. On 6 February, 2015, an arrest was made at Heathrow because the police were out in force in an effort to show commitment to Zero Tolerance of FGM Day, and it looks like it may have paid off.

As they say, 'It takes a village.' Even if people in traditionally practising communities find it difficult to speak out, they still have a duty to do so. Every little bit helps.

My aim is to build with others a World Portal on FGM resources for eradication, with online and archived in print collections, updated daily.

I believe global activism and international federating efforts now require fully-fledged funding. This means we must go beyond the paradigm of 'sincere volunteerism and *ad hoc* donations'. We must refocus assertively to shape a movement that secures synchronised and multi-faceted national and international government funding for the fight against FGM.

We need to get past the puffery and demand that people really care.

....

Our brief survey of activists against FGM in North America demonstrates well, as we saw also in Australia, that several different campaign emphases are developing. Some people focus on what is happening in traditionally practising countries, and some concentrate on FGM in the Western locations to which refugees and others in the diaspora have travelled in search of a new life.

As we have also seen, some activists attend to both aspects of campaigning. More news of developments in all these #EndFGM endeavours can be found on the Female Mutilation Worldwide website. It will be particularly interesting to watch progress in, and perhaps even support, the domestic American and Canadian lobby, as more people understand that FGM is a challenge for North Americans just as it is for those elsewhere.

Now, however, we move on to Europe, where there is probably a more developed awareness of the realities of FGM and, in some cases, significant public efforts are being made to confront these realities.

CHAPTER 8:

Continental Europe

It is thought that about half a million women and girls in Europe have undergone female genital mutilation. Nonetheless, as the narratives in this chapter tell us, awareness of FGM is far from uniform across even those parts of continental Europe which host large numbers of people in the diaspora. FGM is illegal, either by inclusion (for instance, as in France) in wider legislation, or expressly, in all parts of the European Union.

We begin with Hazel Barrett's report of the REPLACE 2 research programme about how the wider European context is being studied. Then we move to look at the situation, moving North to South, in Norway, France, Germany and Italy. Next, in addition to Hannah Wettig's contribution on the Middle East (chapter 5) in which she also considers Germany, we have here Tobe Levin's narrative on the situation in that European country and in the United States. We have already considered Spain in Asha Ismail's contribution from Kenya and Greece will be touched on by Hekate Papadaki in the context of the UK, where she now works.

OVERVIEW

Hazel Barrett is a professor and social scientist with extensive research experience of working on gender issues in sub-Saharan Africa and with diaspora groups living in the European Union. Her work is based at the University of Coventry in the UK, and she has been Director of REPLACE 2, a programme funded by the Daphne III programme of the European Commission, which ran until Autumn 2015.

REPLACE 2 represents a radical change to the way female genital mutilation is tackled in the EU, developing a new approach that integrates individual and community behaviour change within a community-based action approach. The REPLACE 2 partners were Coventry University, FORWARD UK and FSAN (the Netherlands), along with CESIE (Italy), APF (Portugal), Gabinet (Spain) and the International Centre for Reproductive Health, Ghent University (Belgium).

In this piece Hazel explains the *Community Readiness to End FGM Index* which has been developed to identify how ready for change to abandon FGM specific practising groups are, focussing particularly on the diaspora communities included in the REPLACE 2 programme.

***

For much of the twentieth century most people in the West thought FGM was a matter only of historical interest. That impression was dispelled for me by my field studies in The Gambia in the 1980s.

Currently, my main way of getting involved in ending FGM is by undertaking high quality, evidence-based research with FGM-affected communities in the EU via the REPLACE programme. I then try to use this research through academic papers, conference presentations, media engagement and briefing policy makers to raise awareness and influence policy and practice. This research has been ongoing since 2010 and has been funded by the European Commission's Daphne III programme.

My research seeks to be culturally sensitive and non-judgemental, not having preconceived ideas, but rather, listening and probing. We have empathy and respect for those involved, but at the same time we challenge the practice. And we try to be realistic about what can be achieved and by whom.

I have been working with various FGM-affected groups including Eritrean and Ethiopian communities in Italy, the Guinea Bissau community in Portugal, Gambian and Senegalese communities in Spain and Somali and Sudanese communities in the Netherlands and UK. We adapt our communication to our various audiences, and we do not use scare tactics and horrible images that make people turn-off from the topic.

Our research has shown that these communities have very subtle differences in their belief systems concerning FGM. The range of rationales is highly complex.

The role of men in perpetuating the practice has however come through very clearly. Although many men stated that FGM is 'women's business' it became quite clear that they condoned the practice and would only marry women who had been cut and so were deemed 'decent' and 'pure'.

What this research has shown is that different FGM-affected communities living in the EU have different belief systems and community enforcement mechanisms.

In most communities, the social norm supporting the undertaking of FGM has adapted and strengthened in the host country. Neither the fact that FGM is illegal in the EU (so too is taking somebody abroad to have it performed), nor the well-known medical impacts of the cutting, are proving a deterrent to FGM in EU countries. Instead, FGM is often seen as an 'identity marker', a way of showing cultural difference from the mainstream.

Combining 'community-based participatory action' methods with 'behavioural change' approaches, our research has developed an innovative methodology to tackle FGM in the EU. This new methodology is known as the REPLACE Approach.

The REPLACE Approach involves working with communities to understand the belief systems concerning FGM and the social norm or pressure that perpetuates the practice. The *REPLACE Community Readiness to End FGM Index* is applied and the community assigned a score based on six different 'domains' or factors. The outcome of this exercise tells us what behaviour and intervention needs to be focussed on, so we can begin the process of challenging and changing the social norms and beliefs that perpetuate FGM within that community.

For some communities, still at a very low level of readiness to end FGM, straightforward awareness raising and community building is the appropriate action. Then, as communities become more open to change, other actions, such as facilitating inter-generational and inter-gender conversations concerning FGM, become necessary.

If communities consider religion as the 'reason' for performing FGM, this view can be challenged. Authoritative, respected figures are asked to stand up and give definitive religious judgements against the practice.

The *REPLACE Community Readiness to End FGM Index* tells us what type of intervention is needed to end FGM in specific communities. At the same time, by being reviewed at regular intervals, the *Index* will indicate if behavioural change is occurring. Hopefully, these interventions will move FGM-affected communities in the EU towards the 'tipping-point', when FGM is no longer an accepted social norm.

In other words, a social norm that supports FGM has then been 'replaced' by one that does not.

For me, change must come from within these communities. Awareness raising without behavioural change support is not effective. Focussing on individual's choices (sharing legal and health information etc) without also targeting communities (the beliefs and customs of the group) is ineffective because the social norm is so entrenched.

In places such as Palermo (Sicily) one challenge is that the FGM-affected women tend to be newly arrived migrants for whom FGM is not the most pressing problem. Because of their migrant status most of the women do not actually 'belong to a community' with identified leaders (or even share customs or language), so it is difficult to establish contact and influence perceptions to ensure that girls will not be harmed.

I also believe it is important to tackle FGM in the traditionally practising countries. Very often pressure to perform FGM is coming from older relatives back in the home country. What has changed, however, is that there is now less acceptance of FGM Type 3 (infibulation / *'pharaonic'* circumcision) as we see a move towards FGM Types 1, 2 and 4.

We must also be aware of a number of other harmful traditional practices (HTPs), such as labia pulling (a form of FGM), 'ironing' of girls' chests, child and early and forced marriage. But even now, FGM remains very common.

Further, some women who speak out have been threatened by members of their families and community. In some cases the police have been involved. FGM is everyone's business, it is child abuse and a serious form of violence against women.

But worryingly there is also a move towards medicalisation, in response to the health messages surrounding FGM. We know that girls living in EU countries are being sent to have the 'operation' in private clinics in the Middle East and Southeast Asia.

Prevention is always better than prosecution!

My research also suggests that services for survivors are very patchy. Many women do not know how or to whom to go for help and advice concerning the physical aspects of FGM. The mental health side is very poorly supported.

I feel very strongly that we should not criminalise survivors of FGM, but need to put into place services to support them physically and mentally. I am nevertheless concerned that the medical implications and legal aspects of FGM have taken centre stage. Although both are really important, we need to challenge belief systems and to change social norms as well.

My message to civic leaders and policy makers everywhere is, therefore, straightforward. Stop this abuse of girls and women. It has no place in the 21st century.

I do feel too that the governments of EU countries need to make clear statements on the legal position of cosmetic genital surgery (CGS), piercing undertaken with consent at tattoo parlours and so on. By allowing CGS (for non-medical reasons) and piercing, governments are undermining the campaign to end FGM.

My research also shows that many FGM-affected communities equate FGM with male circumcision, in terms of a traditional practice. In fact very often the same local word is used to describe both. Many communities cannot understand why it is legal in the EU to perform male circumcision, yet illegal to do FGM. They see this distinction as a form of discrimination against girls and women. The failure to tackle the issue of male circumcision is undermining the fight to end FGM.

....

NORWAY

Norway has had strict legislation against FGM, whether practised domestically or abroad, since 1995.

Ms H is a political scientist and gender activist who now lives in Norway, where there is no clear data on the prevalence of FGM. Whilst still a very young child in her country of birth, Gambia, she experienced female genital mutilation in a traditional ceremony.

Now, 40 years later, Ms H is founder and leader of an organisation working to combat FGM.

***

I am very concerned about achieving an end to female genital mutilation. The developments I would most like to see are:

a telephone hotline to report concerns, help those at risk and advise victims,

clinics to help victims, including reconstructive surgery and psychological support,

information campaigns, including media engagement with the issues,

community engagement, with the involvement of Imams, and of men generally and

an inter-generational approach and role model engagement

I don't know whether FGM is becoming less frequent in the communities I work with, but I think mainstream society must be active in stopping FGM, along with the traditionally practising communities themselves. Unfortunately, people in these traditional communities do still find it difficult to speak out, because it is taboo to discuss FGM, which is their cultural heritage.

Everyone needs to know FGM is a serious human rights violation that removes a part of the individuals who experience it. Decision makers in the countries concerned must take the fight against FGM seriously and put in place laws and funds to fight its eradication.

Funding is important and so is media engagement. If people in the wider community want to support our work, one good way is to help raise vital funds.

When the eradication of FGM has been achieved, the physical and mental health of a huge number of women and children in the future will be greatly improved.

I don't think male circumcision (male genital mutilation, or MGM) is a topic to be considered alongside FGM.

....

FRANCE

France, where considerably more than 50,000 women are thought to have FGM, has strict general legislation against harm to children The acivitists we meet here focus on the legal system and on health care.

Linda Weil-Curiel, a French attorney, is a distinguished member of the Paris Bar. Her focus is human rights. Over the years she has secured many dozens of prosecutions for FGM, establishing that those suspected of these crimes must be tried in the highest courts, where punishments are severe. Ms E is a British-born lawyer also living and working in Paris, France. She is also a lecturer in law as it relates to FGM and, like Linda Weil-Curiel, makes it clear that her concern is primarily the human rights of the child.

Pierre Foldes, a French citizen, is a urological surgeon working in Paris. He is President of the *Institut en Santé Génésique* (Institute for Reproductive Health, which he founded five years ago with Frederique Martz) and a leading pioneer in post-FGM clitoral reconstruction, which he has provided on a *pro bono* basis for almost five thousand FGM survivors.

For the summer of 2015 Kaillie Winston, an American student, was an intern in Paris, working with the anti-FGM campaigners lawyer Lorraine Koonce-Farahmand and academic Tobe Levin to support Dr Foldes' *Clitoris Restoration Fund* project.

***

Linda Weil-Curiel

I am a French lawyer working in Paris, born in Tahiti. My mother is Polynesian.

Years ago I read in the French press that a baby had died of haemorrhage after undergoing FGM, and that the parents were to be prosecuted for not going to hospital to seek medical help for their daughter. It was in 1982 and another case was also at that time being brought to the attention of the courts. Mercifully, however, the second child survived, thanks to the doctors of Hospital Saint-Vincent de Paul in Paris.

I decided to step into the legal proceedings because the prosecution was based on 'bodily harm' and I thought it should be '*mutilation*', meaning 'grievous bodily harm'. In France, the latter would be a serious crime and can only be brought before the Assizes Court, the highest criminal court, which of course would have been the case with grievous bodily harm if the child were white.

In France we refer to FGM as 'sexual mutilation' rather than 'genital mutilation', to make the point that it is a direct attack on a woman's entitlement and human right to enjoy adult sexual experience.

I still work as a *pro bono* lawyer but I also manage the *Commission pour l'Abolition des Mutilations Sexuelles* (CAMS), founded by Awa Thiam, the author of *Speak Out, Black Sisters: black women and oppression in Black Africa* (1986, translated by Dorothy Blair).

To begin campaigning against FGM, back in the early 1990s, CAMS (meaning in reality my own pocket...) produced the film *Bintou in Paris*, in which a young mother is persuaded to resist her husband's and mother-in-law's demand to have her baby girl excised. This fifteen-minute fictional documentary examines the traditional social pressures put on women to permit FGM on their daughters and was very much appreciated by mothers. The film has English subtitles.

We also developed other campaigning products. The Malian Bamako-born reggae singer Bafing Kul made his first CD, *Exciser c'est pas bon, exciser c'est mutiler* ('Excision is not good, it's mutilation'). T-shirts were produced under the label *Mélodies du Monde* (with Bafing in charge) and I devised a comic strip for the CAMS website. I even wrote a song, *Little Girls from Africa*.

Awareness in Paris and the suburbs has grown in recent decades, and from 1984 onwards health professionals began to tell families why they must not practise FGM. We also call their attention to the fact that FGM is illegal in France, so parents risk being tried and sent to prison if their child is found mutilated. The focus is consistently on the right of the child to remain intact.

We know for sure, because the mothers say so, that the risk of trial has been a deterrent. Information and repression must go together; they are two faces of the same coin. Experience has shown that one without the other is useless.

But when a child has actually undergone FGM, a person with a role like the UK's *guardian ad litem* is appointed by the enquiring judge in the proceedings, which lead to a trial. This person's sole responsibility is to represent the interests of the child quite separately from all other considerations. If FGM is then found to have been committed by the accused, those responsible are required to pay compensation directly to the victim, and the guardian becomes responsible for ensuring this money is kept safe for the girl to receive when she reaches adulthood.

People are not stupid: they understand perfectly that when you cross the line you must expect to be punished. We have seen that 'soft' sentencing is perceived in the relevant communities to suggest tolerance of 'culture' and 'tradition'. A significant level of punishment is necessary to instil an understanding that FGM is never acceptable.

I strongly believe too that the threat of financial sanctions would be a very efficient deterrent.

Social benefits (rather generous in France) should be managed by social services whenever children are at risk of, or have undergone, FGM or 'forced marriage' (in truth, rape). Social benefits should not in those circumstances be handed to the family, because the money should be used in the sole interest of the child, and we very well know that, if these families manage the benefits, that is not always the case.

In France we have populations from the former colonies, mainly West African countries such as Mali, Mauritania, Ivory Coast, Senegal, Guinea Conakry and similar regions, but recently it seems that Egyptian families are also arriving in numbers.

There are fewer East Africans here as they are not French speaking. With all the efforts to stop it, I believe that FGM is now becoming less common in the relevant communities in France.

The state nonetheless still has a major role to play. Social services, doctors, police, judges and prosecutors must be trained in order to detect and analyse properly the dangers to which the girls are exposed. I explained this to a UK audience in 2014 when I was a key witness during the House of Commons Home Affairs Committee inquiry into the lack of prosecutions.

There is no reason for families to resist the physical examinations to which children (boys and girls) up to the school entry age of six are entitled, and this practice is also effective in protecting small girls from FGM. The examinations are not compulsory, but it is unheard of for parents to refuse this opportunity to check on their child's health and development. Medical colleagues who conduct these examinations have confirmed to me that parents know, and acknowledge to the doctor, that evidence of harm will, without exception, be reported.

Also, of course, it is important for the populations themselves to accept that if they reside in a foreign country, they have to adapt, not only because they receive benefits but because their children's future is European.

The children of immigrants won't live the same life as their parents have lived in the country of origin. Customs must be questioned and sometimes put aside, just as the traditional bodily scarification and tattoos are abandoned when people arrive in Europe. These can be seen on the face, and the relevant populations became ashamed of the marks. Evidence of FGM is safely hidden in the knickers, but that practice too must become a matter of shame, and must stop.

The veil is a very oppressive garment, symbolising the aggressive control of women. I cannot support its use in the public realm in Western society, rather as, even more fundamentally, I will never accept FGM conducted in the privacy of the home. Both are designed to make women submissive and obeying. The female body is deemed disturbing for men and they demand it must be hidden. The veil in public space, whatever its size, symbolises the walls of the house, where, in traditional thinking, women should remain.

Likewise, importantly, 'forced marriage' should be re-named as 'rape organised by the parents' and be punished as such. No child or teenager should undergo FGM and no child should be sold, to be regarded as 'married', when in fact she has been a victim of an organised crime - forced marriage - which is forbidden in European countries.

***

Ms E

I first became aware of female genital mutilation about a decade ago, as a law student. Although I have neither witnessed nor experienced FGM, I am a committed campaigner and lecturer against it. It still upsets me and makes me want to cry with sadness and often with frustration.

The judiciary system is a critical part of making FGM history. The message must be clear that FGM is against the law and, when performed or if about to be performed, it is legally punishable. France has a very strong track record and support system in this respect.

I believe that the communities in France are aware that FGM is not legal in France. It is the threat of legal punishment that may be a factor that is helping to eradicate FGM.

Like forced marriage, FGM is a societal problem that everyone needs to speak about and condemn. Perhaps talking about the external female genitals can be uncomfortable for some members of FGM practising communities, but by addressing FGM at the grassroots level as well as the legal level, we can reach the African communities that practise FGM clandestinely.

Obstetric fistula resulting from FGM is a serious problem, and France provides FGM reconstructive surgery to help survivors who want that.

Mutilation is mutilation, but FGM is nonetheless different is some respects from male circumcision. If men's penises were routinely subjected to similar degrees of cutting, a debate about whether we should tackle FGM would not even take place.

We must remember however that, for many African women, marriage is their only means of economic survival. This has to change. Currently, some men will not marry women unless they are cut, so FGM becomes a tool for survival.

I'd suggest that countries where FGM is traditionally practised should demonstrate beyond words their commitment to eradicating FGM before they are given economic aid.

From the depths of my soul, I find that FGM is wrong.

***

Pierre Foldes

I first came across female genital mutilation whilst in Burkina Faso, during a surgical mission in Africa 30 years ago.

As a surgeon specialising in urology I was keen to do something to help women with FGM, and I have subsequently developed a surgical method for reconstructing the clitoris. This method can be applied whatever type of FGM a patient has undergone.

Over the past 25 years I have met more than 15,000 victims of FGM for clinical consultations, and have performed operation for reconstruction on approaching 5,000 women. I continue to do about 50 operations every month.

Five years ago, I met Frédérique Martz. Our common values and our shared concept of work around concern and respect for women victims of any sort of violence, have enabled us to envision a programme to support them.

Together we created our institute, *l'Institut en Santé génésique* (the Institute of Reproductive Health), located in a suburb of Paris. It is a charitable foundation inspired by people we have met in countries where violence is ever present.

The Institute is a pilot project. We are involved in many missions and actions against FGM in Mali, Burkina Faso, the Ivory Coast and Sénégal, and we are part of many campaigns and collective actions.

We are concerned about the growing number of FGM cases in France, and about the evidence that these victims also suffer from other kinds of violence.

The Institute has a team of 26 professional volunteers, directed by Frédérique Martz, and we are developing in-depth knowledge and expertise. We have gathered together doctors, nurses, jurists, psychologists and others, all working *pro bono*, who welcome our patients and offer holistic management of treatment for victims of any kind of violence, including FGM.

We created and enhanced the concept of 'talking groups', gathering in one session women with experience of any kind of violence, including FGM. These meetings help the victims to build a common language and share their different healing processes. The women send a strong message to civil society, showing their adroitness in the face of adversity – a rare and wonderful moment of hope and solidarity.

Through these programmes we also seek to expose and explain the clinical realty of FGM and its consequences. We explain in detail to each patient what type of FGM she has, and we encourage the patient to talk and explore what has happened to her.

It is vital that we listen carefully when victims discuss these matters. FGM (often referred to in the clinic as *'l'excision'*) is an act of criminal violence with many traumatic impacts physically, obstetrically, psychologically, intellectually and socially. With the patient, we explore issues around her privacy, possible treatments (including whether or not she should opt for surgery), work, family and any other concerns she may have.

When all these elements have been fully acknowledged we can progress towards a suitable, tailor-made care pathway for the person concerned.

Importantly, in another regard, the holistic management we provide allows the victims, whether or not they elect for surgical reconstruction, to talk openly about FGM and to bear witness in their various communities to the harm it does and the reasons FGM is a criminal act.

Some of the surgeons and other clinical staff who have trained with us now have their own clinics elsewhere, such as teams trained in the Netherlands, the United States, Senegal, Mali, Burkina Faso and Benin, as well as in other parts of France. Through these teams we spread the word that action can be taken to help women with FGM.

No woman should be left abandoned, trying to survive unsupported with the devastating impacts of FGM. We want to change that, and, with those of our patients who chose to be activists, to tell everyone that FGM must be stopped.

***

Kaillie Winston

I am an American college student from Ohio Wesleyan University working on the Clitoris Restoration Fund (CRF) in Paris for the summer of 2015. With my blue eyes and blonde hair, people often question what it is about FGM that sparked my interest. It's because I have never experienced this, I respond, merely because I am lucky. There is no other reason. No one chooses which culture he or she will be born into.

If I don't speak up how can I expect this to stop happening to my fellow humans? Americans face issues with racism, but working on the CRF has opened my eyes to the problems that plague other nations on a much deeper, internal level, on a cultural level.

I encounter a diverse cultural spectrum every day. With my head buried in a book, I learn about the women in Burkina Faso, Somalia, Senegal, and many other places enduring the pain of the blade. The fight against FGM is no less traumatic on the streets of Paris. In fact, it becomes more real. Everyone knows about 'l'excision.' The French people whom I have met thus far agree, 'c'est inhumane.'

The journey began in a coffee shop, when I met the attorney with whom I would work, Lorraine Koonce-Farahmand. She told me that we would publicise the Clitoris Restoration Fund. We would send out emails to various organisations about the fund and organa a website for the CRF. Our goal is to gather donations to fund FGM victims to receive clitoris restoration surgery.

Our first stop would be Oxford, England, to meet with Dr Tobe Levin Von Gleichen in order to establish the foundation for the CRF. Next, we would go to Geneva, for the United Nations Human Rights Council Session 29 where Lorraine and others would speak on the panel about the processes and challenges in ending FGM. 'Oh,' she said, 'and read this book.' Lorraine handed me the book *Undoing FGM* (Hubert Prolongeau, 2011). It was in this book that I first truly learned about my comrade on the CRF, the surgeon who repairs FGM victims.

I understood that women undergo this torturous, inhumane crime. I understood too that they want to have repaired that which has been unjustly torn away from them. However, I failed to see Dr Foldes' true motivation for performing this surgery until I read about him in *Undoing FGM*. The sole motive behind his work is empathy.

Reading about Pierre Foldes, I discovered that he has the best possible motives as a human rights advocate. 'Once you understand the amount of real pain,' he says, 'you become an activist looking at the aftermath of crime and begin to transcend the purely academic viewpoint.'

This summer, I have learned that in this line of work – fighting against FGM – our goal is, patiently, to change mindsets over time.

FGM is a cultural problem. It drives deeper into society than racism, through traditional ties. Nearly 3,700 miles away from home, however, I find that FGM is no better or worse than racism. These are all human rights issues and there is no way any one person can fight them alone.

Education is the most vital tool in eliminating global concerns. This is not about preaching our own views, but, rather, listening to other's views. Just like Pierre Foldes, we need to listen and truly empathise before it is possible to change a point of view, one person at a time.

....

GERMANY

It is thought that some 60,000 to 70,000 women in Germany have experienced FGM, and somewhere around 20,000 girls and women there remain at risk of it. FGM is illegal in Germany, whether done at home or abroad.

Tobe Levin, an American who has lived in Germany for many years, and Hannah Wettig, a German-born resident, have both long been engaged in international efforts to stop female genital mutilation. Tobe is an Associate of the Hutchins Center at Harvard University, USA and currently also a Visiting Research Fellow and adviser on FGM at Lady Margaret Hall, University of Oxford, in the UK. A much respected veteran in Europe and the USA of decades in the field of FGM studies, Tobe is an eminent academic and translator who, working also with visual artists and other literary colleagues, in 2009 set up and maintains her own single-topic publishing house, *UnCUT/VOICES* Press, to make the experience of FGM and its consequences known and understood by a global readership. She also has plans to create a charitable organisation to support the work of Dr Pierre Foldes, the surgeon who helps FGM survivors seeking physical and psychological restoration and healing.

Hannah Wettig is the coordinator of the Stop FGM Middle East campaign by the Iraqi-German NGO WADI, which is based in Suleymania, Iraq and Frankfurt, Germany. She first encountered FGM in 1994, in Egypt. Research over the years has however revealed that FGM occurs not only in the Middle East, but also across several parts of Asia. Hannah's remit with Stop FGM now also includes Southeast Asia as well as the campaign's original focus.

Tobe Levin

My activism reaches back almost 40 years. In April 1977 the third issue of the new feminist magazine *EMMA* carried an article by Pauline Caravello called '*Klitorisbeschneidung*' (which translates as 'Clitoridectomy', and which we now know as female genital mutilation). When I read this article, the course of my life changed. The issue moved me to realise I'd become an armchair feminist, whereas this was something that shrieked for action to stop it. I was 29 and a graduate student in Munich.

A movement arose in Germany as basketsful of letters reached *EMMA*'s office. Study groups sprang up, asking what was to be done? Lone African campaigners –Awa Thiam, Edna Adan Ismail, Nawal el Saadawi, Marie Assaad and the Babikar Badri Women's Studies Centre in Omdurman advised. In 1978, the German women physicians' association invited Dr Asma el Dareer to speak. (Dareer would go on to publish the first epidemiological study of FGM in the Sudan, *Woman, Why Do You Weep?*, Zed Books, 1982.)

The national coordination (in Germany) of a network fell to my Munich committee and in 1979 a modest book appeared (I. Braun, T. Levin, A. Schwarzbauer. *Materialien zur Unterstützung von Aktionsgruppen gegen Klitorisbeschneidung/ Documentation for groups against clitoridectomy*.) Afterwards, things petered out.

Then, in 1980, African women met at the U.N. Mid-Decade for Women conference in Copenhagen, where delegates reacted with outrage to Fran Hosken's workshop on FGM. A refugee from Hitler, Hosken (1920–2006) had made it her life's mission to eradicate the practice. She coined the term FGM. She researched, wrote, and lobbied international agencies on the subject.

Hosken was, however, notoriously short on tact, and also anti-male. With few allies even among non-African activists, she might be said to have served as the stereotypical 'white Western feminist' so unwelcomed by many indigenous campaigners.

For some of us however, going away was not an option. In 1982, Awa Thiam invited a small group of us from Germany to join her in Dakar for the inaugural conference of CAMS (*Commission pour l'Abolition des Mutilations Sexuelles* – the Commission for the Abolition of Sexual Mutilation / FGM). The proceedings are recorded in my report, with the provocative title *Solidarische Rassistinnen* (Racist Solidarity?) (*EMMA*, February 1983, p.63).

A year later, in April 1983, *Terre des Femmes* in return invited Awa Thiam to address their first annual meeting, in Frankfurt. Shortly afterwards Thiam, the late Efua Dorkenoo, who had just founded the anti-FGM organisation, FORWARD, and a small group from Germany met in Paris to explore how we could work together, given that the issue was viewed as urgent by only a tiny trans-national minority.

An enormous and powerful majority tenaciously then defended, and still defends, the practice of FGM.

Eleven years later, in 1988, I co-founded FORWARD-Germany. Leading up to this point had been work since 1977, supporting African activists, giving speeches and publishing popular and scholarly articles. As one example, I co-edited a special issue of *Feminist Europa: Review of Books* on books about FGM (2010). This work continues, with more of the same. Networking is important, and I now do this principally with the EuroNet FGM founded by, among others, the survivor, Khady Koita – a campaigner very much worth supporting.

Khady in turn inspired the founding of my single-focus publishing house, *UnCUT/ VOICES Press* in 2009. The purpose of this press is to draw greater attention to the experience and impacts of FGM, often by featuring the words of survivors. I also have a website, and have translated numerous articles and documents into English, to ensure they reach a wider readership.

There are many challenges in confronting FGM and problems also of other forms of violence against women, such as breast ironing, heightened danger of fistula in impregnated early teens and children, and the special case of FGM as grounds for asylum, an option pioneered in the early 90s as recorded in Pratibha Parmar and Alice Walker's film *Warrior Marks* (1993).

There is the question of how to achieve reparation (physical, financial, social, etc...) for FGM survivors, including access to reconstructive surgery (I translated and wrote the Afterword to *Undoing FGM. Pierre Foldes, the Surgeon Who Restores the Clitoris*).

Whilst consensus about impacts is clear, terminology is not so easy. Should the words we use censure, blame, persuade, exhort, insult, cajole, seduce, emote – or entertain? Most writers concur with the IAC (Inter-African Committee) on *Traditional Practices Affecting the Health of Women and Children*, whose *Bamako Declaration* of 2005 promotes the rationale for hard, formal terminology.

Others do not, rejecting the word 'mutilation' in favour of 'softer' labels for the harsh realities. These choices inevitably comprise a challenge for the wider debate. I have discussed this in the context of what I call 'Anthr/Apology'.

The discourse becomes yet more complex when we consider the word 'circumcision'.

There are the controversies – especially difficult in nations such as Germany – over male 'circumcision', which I have come to regard as genital mutilation. People need to inform themselves about the physiology of the penis and the harm of which I have become convinced follows from circumcision. As I argued in my 2014 lecture on Genital Autonomy, like FGM, male genital mutilation (MGM) is a clear violation of the child's rights. That is not to say however that the issues can be approached in exactly the same way as FGM.

Regarding cosmetic genital surgery, it has been my opinion that, although it is clearly chosen by women to be fashionably attractive to men, and hence is motivated by hypothesised male desires, because women over the age of majority are doing the choosing, it is my view that they should be permitted to do so.

So what are the ways forward?

Responding here with what I believe the young firebrands like Leyla Hussein and co-campaigners might say, the answer has got to be education, publicity and accountability.

As resident in Germany, I'd like to see the nation adopt measures against FGM as in France, where they have put up the funds for all small children to include routine medical, including genital, examinations.

I want adoption of the Dutch approach, which would be certificates noting the exit of German residents from high prevalence African countries, when they leave and enter Germany with girls of an age to be excised.

I'd like to see as concerted a media campaign in Germany such as *The Guardian* has launched (2014) in the UK and then via the United Nations, in the USA, Kenya and Gambia. The success of this campaign was acknowledged when it was selected as first-prize-winner in the Editorial Campaign category of the 2015 *British Media Awards*. Let's replicate it elsewhere.

Most important to me personally, I'd like to see the universities, especially the African Studies and Women's Studies Departments, finally showing the courage to address FGM.

The battle had not been won. Even in September 2007, for instance, the government in Sierra Leone, where more than 90 per cent of females are cut, was offering as a pre-election sweetener to pay for female teens to have their clitoris and labia minora cut off 'at no cost to their families'. In Freetown, Dr Irene Koso-Thomas, a solitary voice against FGM since 1988, faces as much, if not more, opposition now as ever.

FGM hasn't happened to me personally, except in a broad but applicable sense that I'll explain with the following anecdote, and which perhaps explains in a way why some 'intact' women feel so strongly for those who have endured FGM as such:

Once in the early 90s while browsing shelves in a London bookstore I felt a title spring out at me. The book was called *Painful Sex*. Taking it from the shelf I was thinking, 'At last. Another volume to join the handful to date that have been published on FGM.'

The book was not, however, about FGM, but about dyspareunia, the well-guarded secret that my generation, having benefited from the sexual revolution, suffered from distress in sex. The volume showed, if I remember correctly, that 40 per cent of women (Western of course – taken for granted) were experiencing, well, painful sex – without having had any form of FGM whatsoever.

This reminds me of Nawal el Saadawi's famous comparison in *Daughter of Eve*. Noting that Marie Bonaparte subjected herself to a kind of FGM (to move her clitoris) and that Freud insisted on 'shifting' clitoral pleasure to the vagina, Nawal el Saadawi wrote that Western women undergo psychological clitoridectomy and that the intention of males in societies that cut, and those that normally don't, are thus the same – in both cases to disempower women.

Hence, the taboo about mentioning FGM, because of the taboo about mentioning sex strongly resembles the taboo on mentioning 'painful sex' in a supposedly sexually-liberated society. ... And I can't help throwing an illustration in here. I have a postcard-style photo now under a refrigerator magnet: The man is saying to his (perhaps?) wife, 'Honey, whisper something dirty in my ear'... to which she replies, 'Kitchen?'

As long as sex is dirty, anthr/apologists will be able to claim that seemingly beneficent parents only want the best, that is, to 'purify' their daughters, to make them marriageable. The claim will be made that parents wish simply to delete what is underneath this association of sexuality and dirt, namely male fear.

Beyond that truth and fear, Linda Weil-Curiel (above) has the best grip on it all. If white girls were being chopped up, there would have been a brouhaha long ago. Allowing this to continue is the surest sign of racist indifference and contempt.

....

ITALY

Details of the prevalence of FGM in Italy are only beginning to be available, but recognistion of the problem is growing, especially as more people from traditionally practising countries make their home there.

Valentina Acava Mmaka

Valentina Acava Mmaka, an Italian by birth, currently lives between Kenya, South Africa and Europe. She is a literary writer, creative artist, journalist and human rights activist and, like some others, she has developed a focus on story telling as a way to support FGM survivors and bring issues around female genital mutilation to public attention.

***

I'm a writer so I support the EndFGM cause through art, mainly writing and theatre. I first became aware of female genital mutilation in the mid-1990s, when I heard the writer and activist Nawal el Sadaawi speak about it. Since then, following on from a social theatre project I did in Mombasa, I wrote a play called *Wapi Mama?* (literally *Where Mama?*) where I mentioned the experience of FGM, as I also did in my three monologue plays, *I...immigrant...woman...*, which were widely staged in Europe and Africa and published in Italy by EMI in 2004.

Later, whilst working in Cape Town in 2011, I formed a collective of women called the Gugu Women Lab, where members of the group from Kenya, Senegal, Somalia, Nigeria, Angola and Egypt, also chose to explore their experiences of female genital mutilation. We devised a performance, *The Cut*, from these stories, to raise awareness and create a space and language that could 'give' permission, should they feel they needed that, for other women also to openly talk about FGM.

I've toured in Europe presenting this performance, speaking in schools, associations, communities and readerships. Amnesty International supported the performance for its power in raising awareness on FGM through art. I then wrote a workshop book about my experience (published in Italian, English and French in 2015). I aim to present workshops for students, educators and artist colleagues, starting with *The Cut*.

And there are also other harmful practices that are very rarely spoken of. One of these is so-called 'breast ironing'. Mainly practised in Cameroon, Ivory Coast and Benin, it is done with the hope it will prevent early marriage and 'protect' girls from sexual assault.

There's still a lot of work for us to do.

In South Africa, FGM is practiced by the Venda people, and by immigrants from other African countries where they have already been cut as small children. FGM remains a taboo.

South African immigrants from FGM countries do not speak about it openly, nor does the media represent their reality. This is exacerbated by the stigma which surrounds the whole matter. From an external perspective FGM is condemned, and immigrants who believe in it feel they will be judged if they talk about their feelings and thoughts.

Also, I've observed that FGM has significantly different impact on women's lives in different places. Tackling and improving ways to eradicate it should take these differences into consideration.

For example, in Southeast Asia, where a matter like normal sexuality doesn't have a public language or public space to be discussed in, it seems impossible to talk about FGM. (To illustrate the point, FGM in this part of the world is pretty much unrecognised further afield.) It follows from this that strategies for anti-FGM intervention should be different and somehow brought gradually from a very narrow plane to wider public awareness.

Likewise in Italy FGM is completely a taboo. The media is silent unless someone has died of FGM. Though Italy has one of the smallest numbers of girls undergoing FGM (3,000 to 3,500 per year, though this may rise with more immigration), it is an urgent issue, especially if we relate it to the lack of services such as health care and legal assistance.

I would also like to underline a point about the World Health Organisation (WHO), which is supposed to create awareness about FGM via large institutions. The majority of NGOs are funded by Western capitals, run by Western people, counting on Western volunteers ... this doesn't make much sense in terms of meaningful scale.

Countries like the African ones, where it is mainly smaller organisations which provide the educational tools for FGM practicing communities, should change their approach and see these relatively small NGOs as genuine partners, rather than favouring just the larger institutions which currently fill 90 per cent of the field.

Governments should invest their own money to promote education and information. They should provide the right services, train professionals and involve their own volunteers and business people to invest in social projects. Taking greater responsibility for the issues will lead to a more efficient awareness about the need to change culture and traditions, through the involvement of the whole society. It will make much more sense.

To make sure that FGM will be always spoken about in a liberating and supportive way, I've also started an initiative called the FGM Narrative Workshop which aims to be an ideal virtual and physical creative space whereby to connect people who have undergone FGM and those who haven't, collecting their narratives for the future post-FGM generation.

Society transforms itself continuously. It's essential to prepare generations for global changes on a small and bigger scale. Schools should include FGM and human rights as part of their curriculum, for example through art (theatre, spoken word, music, screenplay, literature) that could increase opportunities for correct and open public dialogue on FGM.

Unfortunately in general this support has not shown up. There's a lot of fear that such moves might not be seen as appropriate, or in some irresponsible cases it's not considered urgent. There's a profound lack of acknowledgement of the impact FGM, not only on survivors or at-risk girls, but also on society as a whole.

To confront FGM we must share stories. Art is an ideal space and tool to connect people's experiences and to convey human rights issues. Its many languages touch the chords of human sensitiveness and it's empathic, so victims of abuse find in art a possible language to express pain, and from there to consider specifics, whether the legal or, for instance, sanitary aspects of the issue in local FGM practicing and immigrant communities.

The diaspora presents quite a challenge. Whilst you might think that confronting issues via a new culture would make people more at ease when discussing delicate topics, there are so many obstacles: the language, not knowing members of other communities, time, basic daily problems (job, legal matters, etc).

Relocating somewhere new does however help us to reconsider our own vision about things (FGM in this case), about our culture, about our beliefs. Migrants could educate their own people that culture is a transformative and mutable experience that is continually enriched. We can give up things which are no longer pertinent, to make room for new experiences.

I wrote and published an open letter to Italian teachers (I've worked there for a long time), offering to help engage the students in issues around FGM, as a delicate and unknown problem. Several educators have, however, expressed to me their fear of bringing this issue into schools, as they think it could become a new way of discriminating against some children.

Nonetheless, I believe keeping young people and families in the darkness and ignorance is a greater form of discrimination. Whether in traditionally practising countries or in some immigrant countries like the USA, young people – boys as well as girls - who have information and tools to recognise FGM as a useless and harmful practice can help to prevent it.

Further into the future, I want people to share stories (in any form) and narratives about FGM experiences, as material for a virtual library. This would be collated from across the world, to be archived when the practice has been eradicated. It will show how FGM had impact on women as well as on men and societies and will enable future generations to see their past with a keener eye.

If they were contributors to such a collaboration, a virtual library could give permission to people who feel reticent today to speak out for the future.

. . . .

In this chapter we have seen increasing pressure, across Europe, to engage public service provision in the fight to combat FGM. Gradually, people in various European countries are grouping together to demand adequate protection for girls at risk, as well as proper care for those who are already victims of FGM. The Female Mutilation Worldwide website will enable us to update on progress in Europe, where reports will be posted on developments and as, for instance for English speakers, more FGM-related material in readers' own languages becomes available. The particular position in the UK, our final destination on this 'global journey', is considered in Chapter 9, which follows.

Chapter 9:

United Kingdom

In Chapter 9, as in the chapters on Kenya and Australia, we consider a single location. Whilst FGM specifically has been illegal in the UK since 1985, it can be argued that it has actually been against the law, as a matter of grievous bodily harm, for much longer than that. The United Kingdom has made some important moves over the past few years to tackle female genital mutilation, not least by tightening up the legislation recently, to include the practice outside the UK and perpetrators who are not British or long-term residents There are thought to be between 130,000 and 170,000 women and girls in the UK who have had, or are at serious risk of, FGM.

Many sorts of people in the UK are working to make FGM history, some of them specifically engaged in campaigns and lobbies, and others professionals in various fields who consciously choose to address FGM in the course of their general business.

The perspectives which various contributors here share as survivors and activists, concerned professionals, people working in policy and so on, offer a comprehensive view of the issues as they are emerging in Britain. In this wider variety of approaches we can discern indications that at last FGM is becoming a mainstream concern, at least in some parts of the UK.

With this range of approaches in mind, Chapter 9 is divided into two sections. Firstly, we consider people whose work is directly about ending and/or repairing the damage of FGM. Most of these people are to be found in the voluntary sector. Some, including a number of survivors, are taking action quite simply as concerned individuals. In the second half of the chapter we turn to others, usually with an already defined wider professional role, who have chosen to develop particular expertise in regard to FGM.

FGM, as many commentators have already told us, will be eradicated only when our community as a whole works to make that happen. The narratives here may prompt ideas about how the many threads could be brought together.

THE SURVIVORS

As they tell us here, survivors react to knowledge of their female genital mutilation differently. There can be no single way to move forward. Possibly most choose or are impelled not to discuss it for some time, if ever. Valentine Nkoyo, a Kenyan from the Maasai community, now lives in Nottingham. She underwent FGM when she was eleven and, after years of avoiding the topic, has now founded a worldwide organisation, the *Mojatu Foundation*, to combat it.

For Ms B, it was more than half a century ago, as an infant in the Yoruba speaking part of Africa that she underwent FGM, but she has discovered only quite recently exactly what happened to her and, like Ms M from Malawi (chapter 4), has until now preferred not to speak about the practice.

Also like Valentine, Virginia Kamara, a qualified nurse and health visitor who has made her home in Coventry, has founded a charity (the *Celestinecelest Community Organisation*, in Coventry). She grew up in South Africa, where she underwent FGM by her father's sister, without her parents' consent.

Other FGM survivors now resident in the UK, whom we have already encountered are Hawa Sesay from Sierra Leone, a social worker and mother of two who lives in Hackney, London, and Hibo Wardere, also London-based and from Somalia (both also chapter 4). They both visit schools and communities to raise awareness, where and whenever they can, of FGM and why it must stop.

***

Valentine Nkoyo

One morning twenty years ago, when I was eleven, my mother told me that I had to become a woman.

She called me by my nickname and said in Maasai, *'Taato, eyiolo ajo etaa kemurati intae?'* meaning *'Do you know it's time you got cut?'*

As per the Maasai culture, I had to be cut. I didn't even know what that meant.

A bull was slaughtered and food and alcohol was in plenty that evening. The entire village thronged our homestead that night to celebrate my 'becoming a woman' in the morning. As they ate and sung, I pretended to be joyful.

But I was terrified. I never slept a wink that night. I didn't know who to talk to, what to say and how to behave. I wanted to run away into the dark! But I did not want to be a coward. Where was I to run to anyway? To shame my family? To be the girl who could never get a husband?

Early the next morning, my sister, two other girls and I were escorted by a group of older women to the bushes where the operation was to take place. They all sang happily at the top of their voices. I remember being asked to sit down and one woman sat behind me and tightly held my legs open. The previous night, they had dipped a big axe inside a basin of water to ensure the water was cold enough the next morning. The cold water was poured on me to numb the pain.

I shut my eyes tightly and clenched my teeth not to utter a word or cry as I would be labelled a coward. Then the sharp razor that had been used on my sister was used again to cut through my flesh. The pain was unimaginable. I had never felt anything like that in my entire life before.

After the operation, my sister and I were led to a room where I passed out due to excessive bleeding. Luckily the bleeding was controlled but I was really weak when I regained consciousness. I still don't know for how long I was unconscious. I was in a state of shock for several days and kept getting blackouts.

The following five weeks were full of nightmares of people coming to cut or kill me. After I was cut, I was allocated a woman who looked after me for five weeks until the wound healed. She would wash me and check the wound every day. I hated being washed as it always brought back the distress and up to this day I hate the smell of Dettol (the disinfectant they used to clean the wound) and the sight of a pool of blood, since I saw my own blood that day.

The face of the woman who cut me has never left me to this date. I can still remember the clothes and jewellery she wore that day. For many years, I avoided any conversations related to FGM as it was so painful to revisit what happened, but stories in the news and on social media made me realise that I cannot run away from what happened to me and that, unless I face the issue of FGM directly, I will never be able to move on.

A year or two ago, my mother rang me from Kenya to let me know that our last-born brother was going to be circumcised. I asked her if she was going to cut the girls (my nieces) too. She asked me to speak to my brother and sisters about it.

After long conversations over a whole year, educating them on the consequences of FGM, my two sisters and brother vowed to never to cut their daughters. One of my sisters was shocked to learn that some of the complications she had gone through were as a result of FGM. All my great-great-grandmothers, great-grandmothers, grandmothers, mother, aunties and sisters were cut.

Sex and FGM are a taboo and a very uncomfortable subject to discuss for many people in the Maasai community, but I could not keep quiet and watch my beautiful nieces have their 'lives cut away'. Winning this argument made me believe that we can actually end FGM in a generation.

Now thirty years old, I am a survivor of female genital mutilation, and in a serious relationship. I would really love to have children. If I am blessed with daughters, *they will never be cut.*

I moved to Nottingham in March 2014, where I am very involved in campaigns against

FGM. I have mobilised survivors, practising communities, the local authority, the police, NHS and organisations supporting women. There wasn't much happening before about FGM in Nottingham apart from big one-off events arranged by organisations from outside Nottingham.

Local survivors and practising communities were not engaged, but now we have a Nottingham FGM Steering Group in place with over 25 countries represented. The majority of them are survivors and individuals from practising communities, plus faith leaders and young people among others. We work with people from Kenya, Ethiopia, Eritrea, Sudan, Somalia, Gambia, Tanzania, Uganda, Nigeria, Sierra Leone, Egypt and Senegal among others.

I have since spoken to conferences across the UK, been on local and national radio stations and spoken in schools and to health and other professionals, bringing to life the reality of FGM and how it's affecting real people.

We have received some support for our general work in Nottingham from the council and the police, but we would benefit with more support from the NHS and other women's organisations. We also need support to set up a survivors' centre so that they don't have to live in isolation. Most importantly, funding the grassroots organisations doing work around FGM will give activists confidence and experience to tackle the problem.

I have not only myself suffered FGM, but there are other issues I have had to face as a young Maasai Woman. I was sexually abused by drunkards and I didn't know what to say or where to go for help. Some of FGM survivors are actually also survivors of other forms of abuse and their troubles therefore run deeper than the issues they share with the public.

There are other harmful practices like child marriage (I escaped this myself) and also discrimination when it comes to education. I was not given equal education opportunities compared to my brothers. I was criticised for asking to be educated. Even issues around inheritance of property especially among the African communities has been an issue. Boys inherit but girls don't in certain communities.

I love Kenya, my country of origin, and I want leaders there to make the law work and prosecute those who break it. Individuals, including politicians and other educated people, who advocate for FGM should face the full force of the law. Others can help us by supporting those championing against the practice.

Being connected to other campaigners taking part in this book and sharing opportunities is a fantastic idea. I wish Hilary and all my co-narrators the very best of luck.

***

Ms B

I am in my late fifties and have lived in Britain for a long time. However, I was born in the Yoruba speaking area of West Africa. I underwent female genital mutilation when I was just a baby, but obviously I can't recall how it was done.

I sort of knew from childhood. A maid checked me and a female cousin of similar age when we were about four, but I didn't know the connotations or details.

My father was probably away on business when the procedure was performed. He paid for the operation to manage matters. I suspect he would not have approved and was presented with a *fait accompli*. He may even not have known until I had to have the 'operation'.

I guess even back then not many educated people of their generation would have mutilated their daughters. My mother was herself educated and had me late in life, so, in my thinking, she should have known better; but she was never forthcoming about anything, so if I had actually asked her about it she would not have responded. Unfortunately therefore I was never able to explore the reasoning with her.

In terms of physical aspects, some of my core muscles are compromised, which has affected my enjoyment of activities such as dance (which I had to give up) and yoga. I am now more aware of these impediments, so I am working on them. The compromised core muscles also impact on various other activities. Being improperly balanced affects posture and diaphragm and breathing.

Recently raised awareness of the connections between FGM and my body also means I am constantly readjusting myself, particularly when seated. This could well be as a result of a surgical intervention in my twenties interfering with the 'pull up' of pelvic floor muscles.

And sex has always been a problem. I choose not to look for it, unlike many others who seem to seek it out. I am bitter, as I believe FGM impacted negatively on the prospects for my having a fulfilling relationship and family. I have no children though I have been married. I have mainly been without partners and would find it hard, no that my awareness has been raised, to enter into any such relationship. I am reluctantly resigning myself to a companionless life.

The personal impacts of FGM are lifelong, both physically and psychologically.

This 'procedure' is a horrid mutilation and secret, with lifelong consequences for physical and psychological well-being and my self-esteem. It's something I would never want anyone to know about me - some do know, and have gossiped. I have been mortified. I feel defective.

It is likely that the pain of the early FGM also triggered pre-speech trauma, creating significant issues which continue despite several psychoanalytic and other interventions. Recently I have focussed on time-line analysis, which has had some effect, but I still struggle.

I have really only internalised, and increasingly understood about, FGM in the past few years, despite having had to have a surgical intervention to facilitate sexual activity in the second half of my twenties.

I don't really get involved directly in campaigns against FGM, so I am still quite 'new' to considering wider aspects of FGM, only recently having had my FGM II status confirmed by Comfort Momoh, when I took a trip to her clinic. It has taken me a while to develop a view, not due to the difficulty or otherwise of the subject matter, but due to disinclination resulting from my mental ill health, which may be partially due to the effects on relationships and so on of having undergone this procedure.

Some ways forward in addressing the general issues do however come to mind. I am aware that many, like myself, would not like to be identified, so workshop formats may be difficult, but what would be helpful would be practical information and help.

It would be great if there could be:

- workshops raising awareness and giving information on what can be done to improve quality of life, both psychological and physiological,
- surgery improving physical comfort and the sexual experience,
- targeted psychotherapy and
- targeted exercise classes to improve posture, walking and breathing.

Whilst I am not familiar with any of the communities still practising FGM, I would say education, and empowerment of the female so they can think through consequences themselves, are required. Like parenting, these are things that should be taught from very early childhood. Skills for commitment, nurturing and general human rights are needed by everyone and would also help eradicate FGM.

Wherever it occurs in the world mainstream society should also be active in stopping FGM. I believe in the global community but understand that this could be culturally sensitive – how far will interventions to stop FGM be seen as cultural imperialism?

***

Virginia Kamara

I live in England now, but I grew up in South Africa. My parents allowed my paternal aunt to take care of me because she couldn't conceive children of her own, but they kept my five sisters at home with them. The upshot was that I underwent female genital mutilation, but my sisters didn't.

FGM skipped my mother's generation as my grandmother believed it was irrelevant and that it didn't carry any benefits for girls and women. My paternal aunt however had other views, and she and her friend performed FGM on me, systematically and intrusively, when I was aged somewhere between five and nine.

My biological parents were not aware of what my aunty was doing. After they found out there was total family breakdown and no further contact with the paternal side of my family.

Years later, I myself have children. My daughter was the first person to whom I explained in full what happened to me.

I am a qualified nurse and health visitor, and the founder of the Celestinecelest Community Organisation based in Coventry. Celestinecelest is a not for profit organisation founded in 2013. Our aim is to raise awareness of female genital mutilation. Locally, nationally and internationally we are a vocal prosecutor for FGM. We believe that female genital mutilation is an act of misogyny, violence against women and children, and a violation of human rights.

I participated in the first Coventry FGM concert and have conducted workshops and participated (so far) in two FGM research projects. I conduct home visits and discussion forums on FGM, safeguarding, child marriage and forced labour and I raise awareness about the benefits of a healthy sex life, including raising awareness of HIV/AIDS, chlamydia, gonorrhoea and hepatitis A, B and C plus contraception.

Although my allies and I are serious about our task, our way of communicating and approach to sexual health is not understood. We are experts in this subject, but we are not supported financially and most of us struggle as voluntary groups. Professionals would rather refer to big organisations, but these agencies don't have pathways to manage our specific needs.

There must be recognition and financial support for voluntary services to end FGM that are run and operated by African communities. It is time to stop using them to justify grants received by big organisations that claim they support voluntary organisations through booking a hall and buying refreshments. We are the ones who have access to our communities, but we never seem to qualify for funding.

Most practitioners out there addressing FGM are not from practising communities. Our communities only see or hear from us, ourselves community members, as activists, not as enforcers of change, because we are only found in the voluntary sector and we are not employed to address FGM. They don't see us as practitioners but as sell-outs.

Our passion is what keeps us going but it doesn't pay for mortgages or basic needs. It is well known in our communities that we are voluntary groups. Once you come out openly against FGM, your whole family is exposed, it is hard and we do lose friends and family.

FGM is abuse and sometimes I feel it is forgotten or taken for granted that we, the survivors, live this day in, day out. Those looking in from the outside should realise that FGM is not just for their dissertations or grant applications, they must have compassion. Please stop telling me you do not understand why a mother does this to her daughter. There are still our mothers. Don't make assumptions that we hate them.

There's little respect and compassion for women when, as adults, they learn from clinicians for the first time that they have undergone FGM. All the literature is about raising awareness of FGM. No one speaks about the difficulties women and men face after all the storm has broken.

African women should be employed in the facilitation of change. It must be accepted that we as African women are entitled to critically appraise FGM service provision pathways, and to suggest other methods, without being made to feel guilty. Please acknowledge that we can support each other and do it effectively, that we want to stop FGM, and that we don't want to be forgotten as soon as we leave a meeting just because we are not big organisations.

For myself, I have discovered that understanding health, policies and procedures, safeguarding and the law can be of a disadvantage in professional contexts, but my experience and skills are appreciated by practising communities themselves.

My perception is that it's OK to speak in conferences where I am labelled a victim and survivor, and it's OK to be grateful that the UK is taking steps in tackling FGM. Where, however, are the women and families who are living with the consequences? Why are African women themselves not in paid positions to address FGM?

There are other awkward questions too: Is deinfibulation working as a provision for women with FGM? How many women who are deinfibulated to give birth are later subjecting themselves to be reinfibulated? What is the difference between an 18-year-old choosing labiaplasty and vaginoplasty, compared to an 18-year-old choosing FGM?

Also, why do people compare FGM and male circumcision? Research has suggested that male circumcision is beneficial to men as it lessen chances of contracting STD's and HIV. When a young boy's foreskin becomes too tight, sometimes it is necessary to circumcise for him for medical reasons. Unfortunately male circumcision cannot be compared to FGM in any way.

FGM is becoming more hidden. Victims are getting younger because of the gaps in services to protect very young children. It's easier to detect that a child is at risk when she is older. We are going to be faced with a crisis of losing girl children because they will be sent back home never to return to the UK until later in life. Some parents have daughters who have had FGM and are still living in Africa. They are now facing dilemmas about bringing their children back to the UK again.

Eradication of FGM will present a better future for women, children and men. Then the NHS and worldwide health organisations can save money and invest it in treating diseases and conditions that are not man-made.

FGM is like a second skin. It is always lurking in the shadows. I can't forget it. I try to live my life the best way I can.

....

Four other UK campaigners against female genital mutilation came to Britain from different parts of the world. Like her medical colleague Phoebe Abe-Okwonga, Sarah McCulloch fled Uganda at a time of political turmoil, and now works to support other women from the diaspora. In 1997 Sarah set up the Agency for Culture and Change Management (ACCM Sheffield, now also ACCM (UK), in Bedford), after learning about female genital mutilation in the Somali community in that city.

Esther Oenga from Kenya, completed her doctoral studies at Reading University and now resides in that town, where she is Chair of the Utulivu Women's Group, a registered charity working to engage local women, children and senior citizens from minority ethnic communities.

Comfort Ottah, a Nigerian by birth, has lived in London for many years. She is a midwife specialising in the support and treatment of women with FGM. In the mid-1990s she served on the board of the anti-FGM charity The Foundation for Women's Health, Research and Development, FORWARD (UK), and was also its managing director. In 1996 Comfort was keynote speaker at the launch of (I) NTACT, the first German NGO devoted entirely to fighting FGM.

Hekate Papadaki was born in Greece and came to the UK over a decade ago, working first as a microbiologist, before moving to the voluntary sector, managing advice and advocacy services for asylum seekers, refugees and migrants. She is now the Grants and Development Manager of the London-based Rosa Fund, a charitable fund set up to support initiatives that benefit women and girls in the UK.

Mayameen Meftahi came to campaign against FGM via a different route. She is a British registered psychotherapist who converted to Islam some years after marriage to her Muslim husband. It was then that she discovered some Muslim women have undergone female genital mutilation, which led her to a close examination of Islamic scriptures. She actively campaigns to persuade other women in her community that the practice of FGM must not continue.

Hekate Papadaki

Hekate Papadaki was born in Greece, and has been living in the UK for the past eleven years. She now works with the London-based Rosa Fund, a charitable fund which supports women and girls.

***

The first time I heard about female genital mutilation was when I read Waris Dirie's book *Desert Flower* as a twelve-year-old girl in Greece, where I was born.

FGM is rarely discussed in Greece, and if it is mentioned, it's mentioned as something that happens 'elsewhere'. Given the rates of migration in the country, however, FGM is undoubtedly an issue that affects many girls and women living in Greece. I am involved with a Greek human rights NGO and I hope to support them to be the first to start the campaign there.

It is harder for people in communities anywhere to speak out in if conversations around FGM are not already ongoing. That's why it's extremely important to support local champions who take a stand against the practice. Local community members who speak out can effect considerably more change in attitudes within their own communities than headlines in national papers.

I have been working with women affected by FGM for the past five years, and since 2013 I have been managing the UK-wide Tackling FGM Initiative at Rosa Fund. The most helpful skills I have learnt over the years are patience, being able to keep calm when people are being offensive or irrational, and always responding with facts and evidence.

In the UK, I first came across FGM in 2008, when I was working for the Manor Gardens Welfare Trust. There, I managed a Bilingual Health Advocacy service for non-English speaking refugees and migrants. One day, I was observing a training session about working in maternity services delivered for our Bilingual Health Advocates. The trainer was discussing the needs of women who have had FGM and the UK law. I overheard two of our female trainees discussing how you had to at least do 'sunna' because it was part of becoming a woman. One of them also said that she had attended a FGM procedure in Harley Street in the 1990s (we reported that but the clinic had since closed).

In my current position at Rosa I work directly with most UK-based organisations working to end FGM as well as with FGM survivors.

The Tackling FGM Initiative is the largest ever UK investment in grassroots FGM prevention work, totalling £2.8 million over six years. The Initiative was founded in 2010 by three independent charitable organisations – Trust for London, the Esmee Fairbairn Foundation and Rosa Fund. At the end of Phase 1 in 2013, the funders were joined by Comic Relief and a central management post was created to drive the strategic impact of the Initiative (this was the post I took on).

Options UK conducted a baseline study of community attitudes around FGM in 2010 and repeated the study in 2013 to assess the impact of the Tackling FGM Initiative. It was found that:

- rejection of FGM has increased where community-based preventive work is taking place,
- funded projects have increased understanding of what works in tackling FGM in the UK,
- working with younger women to empower them to speak out and make

decisions has been more effective than trying to change the often deeply entrenched opinions of older people,

- awareness of FGM is rising, and discussions about FGM are taking place more frequently and
- community groups have a valuable role in comprehensive responses to FGM.

The Tackling FGM Initiative is currently the only network in the UK to combine the wealth of expertise of small grassroots community groups and long-term campaigners in the field of FGM. We seek to communicate what works and what doesn't work in community based prevention with all frontline statutory and voluntary sector organisations across the UK and beyond.

We have also developed a wealth of resources over the past four years including education resources for schools, plays, awareness-raising material, videos, pictures and performances, a lot of which have been shared with the Home Office in the process of developing the resource pack for frontline professionals.

Nonetheless, the campaign can be extremely draining at times. We always have to fight our corner to prove that protecting girls from FGM is important, or that FGM happens in the UK. Attitude change on the ground is very slow.

Despite the growing momentum of the campaign, I can still find myself in community workshops where the majority of participants support the practice and have never heard of the *FGM Act*. Worst of all is the ever-present cultural relativism. Every time I speak in a public forum, there will be someone in the audience who will question our 'interference' in people's 'culture'.

There isn't a single solution to addressing FGM. The Tackling FGM Initiative works with all FGM affected communities and they often have very different justifications for practising FGM. For example, using religious arguments will not be particularly effective with the Kurdish community while it may have a significant impact with the Somali community.

In essence, however, FGM is a practice that stems from gender inequalities and should be addressed as such. In my experience, the most effective approach has been working with young people – girls and boys – to help them understand their rights, address gender stereotypes and help them develop healthy relationships. At the same time, young people need to be supported to engage their families in conversations about ending FGM.

It would be extremely helpful if there was training on FGM in schools and if teachers knew how to identify and protect girls at risk. It would also help if social services knew how to assess the risk of FGM. Unfortunately, they don't.

No risk assessment framework on FGM currently exists which makes it extremely difficult for social workers to intervene to protect girls. Having said that, I'm very pleased at the progress in health services and I'm optimistic that the new reporting and recording requirements will ultimately lead to better understanding of FGM in the UK context and enable professionals to better support survivors and protect girls at risk.

I also believe that male circumcision (or male genital mutilation, MGM) is a cultural practice that must end, although FGM and MGM may need to be tackled separately. Even when MGM is undertaken in healthcare settings by trained professionals, it can still affect sensitivity of the male genitals and should be avoided unless there's a medical justification. I have also spoken to men who were traumatised by the experience, especially in countries where it's practiced on older children rather than babies. At worse, MGM practised in traditional settings by non-qualified circumcisers can have very serious health complications.

The cost of FGM is extremely significant and stifles the potential of millions of women around the world. It is also a practice that cannot be tackled in isolation. It is associated with the oppression of women around the world and it is often a precursor for further abuse including child and forced marriage. FGM does not only compromise the future of the girl upon which it is inflicted but also that of the children born to her.

***

Comfort Ottah

As a Nigerian-born midwife working in London I have attended and delivered many women who have undergone female genital mutilation. My first encounter with FGM was dramatic.

Whilst still a young midwife I was suddenly confronted with the extreme task of delivering an infibulated woman who was screaming, 'Cut it! Cut it!' I felt ready to faint, but I did as instructed. The built up pressure pushed the baby out with such force that the infant and I were thrown back against the wall.

The huge responsibility for lives and deaths encapsulated in that episode left me inwardly trembling, as I pondered what further professional challenges I would be obliged to overcome. I know the harm that FGM causes. I will not accept any reference to it that appears to neglect the impact of this serious intentional injury and abuse.

The fight to establish the hurt of FGM has been going on for decades. Sometimes people refer to it by the euphemism 'female circumcision'. At one point, now years ago, there were even people who defended it overtly. My response in both cases was vehement protest.

In London in 1991 two female African heritage local councillors in the borough of Brent caused quite a stir (having already declared their support for the Ugandan dictator and mass murderer Idi Amin – who had caused thousands of Asian Ugandans to flee the country in fear of their lives) when they demanded that 'female circumcision' be legalised for African families in the UK. (Later, it is said these same two women claimed to be witches who could put spells on dissenters to their policies.)

As footage from the American writer Alice Walker's film *Warrior Marks* demonstrates, the public rally against these Brent councillors' sickening proposals saw me right there, protesting as loudly as I could.

But more was to come. In 1996 I read Harriet A. Washington argue, in the now defunct African American magazine *Emerge*, that 'nearly 60 percent of newborn boys in the United States undergo a similar ritual' to that of girls.

Whilst male circumcision and FGM are now often (in 2015) seen as matters of bodily integrity and human rights, in Washington's treatment the term 'female genital mutilation' became 'a judgmental term that lumps together many types of female circumcision' such as 'clitoridectomy (in which) the clitoris is nicked...'. In response to such trivialisation and its discouragement of action against FGM, in September 1996 I wrote the following letter to the editor of *Emerge*:

Dear Mr George Curry,

[Having] recently read ... Harriet A. Washington on "the rite of female circumcision," I find it offensive and insensitive to the suffering millions of African women and girl children.

How can she compare male circumcision to Female Genital Mutilation? Does she know how many men go out to satisfy their sexual needs because it is impossible with their [genitally mutilated] wives? Does she know how many women are abandoned by their husbands because they shrink away due to pain each time the husbands come near them for sexual relationship? Does she know how many broken marriages there are due to lack of sexual relationship between the man and his wife? Does she know how many men have become impotent simply because each time they approach their wives, they weep with agony? How can you be hurting the woman you love? they ask.

How many babies have died due to obstructed labour? How many women have been left in a morbid state after childbirth due to prolonged obstructed labour and damage to adjacent organs? ...

Does she know how many schoolgirls go off sick every month because they cannot menstruate freely? Does she know how many schoolgirls spend 30-45 minutes trying to pass urine and are always in trouble with their teachers for being late to classes? Does she know how many schoolgirls are expelled from classes because they are described as disruptive and erratic in their mood swings? No one understands what they are going through as they have been sworn to secrecy never to mention their pain and suffering to anyone else.

Does she know how many suffer from recurrent urinary tract infections?

I have met these women and these girls in my daily work both in the community and in the hospitals.

In some African societies, stretching of ear lobes until they reached shoulder length was a culture but ... is now a rarity. Knocking off two front teeth was a culture; ... it is no longer the case today. Tribal marks that deformed the face [were part of] culture in the past; people are now seeking plastic surgery to erase them.

... Killing of twin babies was a culture before but now twins live and are cherished. Binding of feet, chastity belts, burning of widows or burying them alive, denial of voting rights for women, slavery, are cultures (now) past because culture is dynamic and not static ...

... Enough politics (has been played) with the blood, health and rights of African women and their daughters. Enough is enough.

Comfort. I. Ottah, midwife
FORWARD, U.K.

***

Sarah McCulloch

I first learnt about female genital mutilation when I saw a documentary called *Black Bag*, produced by the Foundation for Women's Health Research and Development (FORWARD), a leading African diaspora women's campaign and support organisation with a focus on FGM, child marriage and obstetric fistula.

The film showed that the Somali community in Sheffield were performing FGM, and a Yemeni man was highlighted as the cutter. This made me feel something needed to be done. My main objective then was to establish if this was really happening and what services were available for victims.

I worked closely with FGM survivors, who enabled the project to develop as they told their horror stories and yet lovingly accepting that this was their culture, done out of love and to protect them.

Speaking with survivors the main people involved were the mother, grandmother and maternal aunts (often the mother's sisters), with the cutter being an old woman from the village. In a period of over 15 years I have come across fewer than ten women who said they were cut in a hospital or by a health professional. Of the over 300 women I've talked to, none was cut by a man.

At least 30 per cent of the women said their fathers were against them being cut. Two of these women, sisters, went and had FGM done on themselves due to peer pressure, and 15 years later their father who protected them remains unaware they underwent the procedure.

Some of the survivors have been working with me since 1997, and some have set up their own projects to tackle FGM within their own communities or become Champions or volunteers. ACCM *(UK)* was set up in 2008, although its FGM campaign origins started in Sheffield with the establishment of Agency for Culture and Change Management – ACCM (Sheffield).

Training and raising awareness across all service providers, statutory professionals and the community is also crucial, not only to support victims but also to enable people to understand what FGM is and the ways that it impacts, and how then to work towards its elimination.

Our experience working with victims suggests there should be FGM specialist clinics in every local maternity hospital, with counselling services for every victim. Campaigns should not just concentrate on the girl or women at risk, but also acknowledge that all the women from FGM practising communities are victims and need services, support and respect. They should *not* be treated as perpetrators or called barbaric.

Nonetheless, FGM is becoming less common as the issues come out in the open. Some practitioners no longer do the Type III, but are talking of the 'milder' Type I or Type IV. This is in the right direction though we want them to move to completely end FGM.

Many in the communities we work with say they are not going to use services because they do not want to get themselves or their parents into trouble. They are very fearful of being arrested. Also, FGM is not the 'only' form of harmful traditional practice we see. We know that 'honour' based violence, child, early and forced marriage, and witchcraft are also becoming more common in the UK.

Reliance on activities or agencies who have their own agendas is not helpful. Often communities will just ignore external campaigns, become angry and aggressive. Most importantly, they don't attend externally developed activities or events.

Campaigners from within communities are often targeted and threatened and are seen as traitors. That is why few religious or community leaders speak out.

Yes, if a child is at risk, of course that needs to be reported, but let's help victims – the women who have already undergone FGM – as a first step. Otherwise there is a risk that victims of FGM will be less likely to engage with health professionals, and that leaves their daughters at risk too.

We as campaigners need to accept that this is a deeply ingrained cultural practice that will take a long time to end. Change will come from within the communities themselves as well as from external pressure.

The current very modest funding for grassroots organisations indicates a lack of seriousness about community work to end FGM. Community engagement is seen as an add-on or afterthought, but it is the most important element in campaigns against FGM.

The government's policy of ending FGM in a generation is unrealistic. Any campaign to eliminate FGM will take a long time. In Kenya for example there is a lot of talk about successful prosecutions and setting up refugees and schools for girls, yet in December 2014 whole villages performed FGM openly in defiance of the law!

There are *no* short cuts.

***

Esther Oenga

Female genital mutilation is practiced in Kenya, my country of origin.

December is the month for the 'celebration' by female genital mutilation of young girls aged between six and thirteen years. It is done by traditional female circumcisers who continue to use tools such as razors, and causes long-term psychological pain for survivors. It is a sensitive issue and collective effort is required to fight it at all levels.

The incidence of FGM has decreased drastically due to the awareness of the negative impacts and the government initiatives to stop the practice, but it does still go on in many African communities, particularly in Kenya, where I come from.

I am Chair of the Utulivu Women's Group, which serves Reading, Bracknell, Slough, Wokingham and surrounding areas. ('Utulivu' is a Kiswahili word meaning 'patience'.) Our charity was launched back in 2004 and won a Queen's Award in 2011 for voluntary service. We've organised conferences on themes such as End FGM: This Girl Should Never Be Cut (2014) and End FGM: Zero Tolerance World FGM Day (2015) which have been well attended by teachers, nurses, GPs, solicitors, the Thames Valley police and crime commissioner, politicians, social workers, survivors and others. We addressed FGM from faith, cultural, health, men and survivors perspectives.

FGM survivors need to be supported and individual organisations addressing FGM must work together as partnerships to fight FGM. The perpetrators must be punished for others to learn.

FGM should be a concern for us all. FGM is real, it is happening and I think it will take some time to eradicate. The message is let us not give up, but work together.

***

Mayameen Meftahi

I am British and converted to Islam. I am a registered psychotherapist practitioner and Neuro Linguistic Programming (NLP) life skills coach. I have undertaken professional training in approaches to the prevention of FGM and forced marriage.

I have not experienced female genital mutilation myself. I first learnt about it when I embraced Islam as a British woman a few years ago, after nine years of marriage as a non-Muslim to a Muslim man. I adopted my new faith wholeheartedly, with a strong firm view of 'living Islam correctly', so I began to read about and study particular schools of thoughts and Sharia Law.

During my studies, I came across a very small passage that mentioned female circumcision – what I now call female genital mutilation – as 'sunna', i.e. the way of life prescribed as correct behaviour for Muslims on the basis of the teachings and practices of the Islamic prophet Muhammad (peace be upon him) and interpretations of the Qu'ran.

Having never come across FGM previously, even though my husband is an Arab man, and we had lived in an Arabic country, I was surprised that this was part of my 'religion'.

My surprise was combined with distress because of previous personal experience. The delivery of my first child had involved a very difficult labour and afterwards I had incorrect stitching of the episiotomy and a subsequent haematoma – a very traumatic experience as a wife and a new mother. I then had to undergo further operations to be re-cut and re-stitched in order to continue as I would say 'being a woman'.

Therefore, when I read the passage about FGM I was full of mixed emotions. I couldn't bear the thought of going through something like that again, lifesaving though the original surgery had been. I feared that FGM could be detrimental to the part of my body with which had already had so much trauma.

Being firmly committed to an Islamic lifestyle, I considered whether maybe somewhere there is a justifiable reason for this to take place, but when my husband returned home and I told him about my findings concerning FGM he was in absolute shock and was adamant I didn't need to go through this.

This then is in brief the story of how my journey around FGM began. I needed to put my mind at rest that firstly, I didn't need to undergo this 'procedure' and secondly, I also wasn't compromising my religion by not doing so.

I contacted many organisations around the United Kingdom to start my investigations, as well as researching Islamic sources, trying to fine tooth comb where this particular passage had stemmed from and how authentic it was, given that I know one of the basic principles of Islam comes from Prophet Muhammad (peace be upon him) who said, 'Do not harm yourself or others.'

My findings were that this was a very weak hadith (a hadith is a report of the teachings, deeds and sayings of the Prophet). It has reached us in modern times through un-narrated and uncertain chains of reporting and cannot be fully validated.

I also discovered that FGM pre-dates Islam. Though it may have continued during the time of the revelation of Islam, it was certainly not something Prophet Muhammad (peace be upon him) encouraged, and his wives and daughters were never 'circumcised'. It is also not stated as a requirement in the Qu'ran.

It's now nearly a year since I began my research on FGM, and since I started my campaign and work concerning it. My family and most importantly my husband have fully supported my efforts, especially as I work to educate women in Islam that FGM is not a religious obligation and is in fact contradictory to what is mentioned throughout the Holy Qu'ran. Allah created us in the finest form.

Male circumcision is often performed not just for cultural or religious reasons, but also because of health problems, infections and so on. FGM has no health benefits at all.

So now I work actively as an FGM specialist and trainer. I train professionals, such as my forthcoming training session for our local police officers. As a registered psychotherapist practitioner and life coach, I also work actively within the community, providing a support system for women who have suffered FGM or feel they may be at risk.

The best thing is working with the communities in a sensitive, understanding way. As with any deeply embedded belief, FGM is sometimes a taboo subject that is silenced, but we have to remember that for many communities it is not considered a 'harmful practice'. It's what they have done for generations and for many, it's seen as a protection from rape, honour, status and so on. It's a very complex issue.

I offer talks, courses and life skills workshops to educate people towards eradicating the practice, always careful to be sensitive to the needs and vulnerabilities of those already affected, and their families. I am limited in what I can achieve, however, as my project is completely unfunded.

FGM has become a huge part of my life. It has helped me heal from the trauma I suffered with my first born (though there's no comparison with actual FGM) and if I can give back just a little, then I will continue to do so.

I feel passionately about ending all harmful traditional practices (HTPs), whether FGM, forced marriage, honour-based violence or whatever. My feelings about all HTPs are very complicated, but ultimately FGM takes my heart because of the similar experience I went through. The emotional and psychological impacts were huge.

The vision we all share is a world free of violence to women. People can take the first step by reading about FGM, just as I did. My reading led me to campaign and to dedicate my project to women. Never underestimate what one can do by reading.

....

UK-BASED INTERNATIONAL CAMPAIGNERS

Cath Holland is a British midwife who works in Pokot, Kenya training other clinicians, attending the women in local communities and working to bring female genital mutilation to an end. Cath has founded a charity, Beyond FGM, which operates in Pokot and seeks to prevent FGM, replacing it with Alternative Rites of Passage (ARPs).

Ann-Marie Wilson, a British-born psychologist, founded a values-based charity, 28TooMany, to end FGM. The charity's primary focus is research and enabling local initiatives, particularly in the 28 African countries where FGM is practised, and across the diaspora. The UK remains her working base.

Hazel Barrett is Professor of Development Geography, and Executive Director of the Centre for Communities and Social Justice, at Coventry University, UK. Hazel is also Director of REPLACE 2, a European Commission programme funded by Daphne III, one aspect of which is development in the UK of a mobile phone app to engage young people in issues around FGM.

Cath Holland

I am a British midwife who has practised for some years in Pokot, Kenya, training other clinicians, attending the women in local communities and working to bring female genital mutilation to an end. I run a charity, Beyond FGM, which operates in Pokot and seeks to prevent FGM, replacing it with Alternative Rites of Passage (ARPs).

I first became acutely aware of female genital mutilation as a student midwife, at an Association of Radical Midwives (ARM) conference in the UK, in 1991. The principal speaker was the revered late Efua Dorkenoo whose presentation was on FGM.

A while later, in 1998–2000 I spent two years on Voluntary Service Overseas (VSO) as midwifery tutor in Ortum Mission Hospital School of Nursing in Pokot, Kenya. This is where I encountered FGM on a very personal level, both whilst teaching my students in a clinical setting where the majority of women had undergone FGM, and also in 1998 when I attended the 'ceremony' of my young friend Nellie.

The ceremony was a major community event. The first stage was performed in public where I can only assume that parts of the labia majora were very quickly cut off. I have since heard this described as the clitoris being removed, but this was surely impossible judging by the speed of the cutting.

Some eight or ten girls were cut at the same time, with the same knife, which of course can spread diseases such as HIV/AIDS. Many men were also present, but they faced away, smoking and chatting. They all left after this first stage.

The girls were then led into a secluded bushy area where the rest of the cutting took place. People in Pokot say this stage can take up to five hours, as women inspect the unfortunate girls' genitals and suggest more cutting here and there.

When all the girls had finally been cut they were rested in the open, on beds of leaves. My friend Nellie asked for soda (fizzy drink) which I went to fetch from village. Nellie and her friend wanted me to take photos. (I still have them). After a couple of hours Nellie and her family danced home up the mountain, singing and whistling all the way. There was then a party at home, after which Nellie went into seclusion for about three weeks before a 'coming out' ceremony.

Later, I returned to the UK and in 2005 two Kenyan midwives, Miriam Petakwang and Rhoda Lodio, joined us here and met FGM specialist clinicians such as Dorcas Akeju

OBE (Liverpool Women's Hospital FGM specialist midwife, a founder of the UK FGM Clinical Group), Dr Jo Topping (a Liverpool Women's Hospital consultant obstetrician) and Comfort Momoh, FGM specialist midwife at Guys' and St. Thomas' Hospital in London, as well as the FGM activist Leyla Hussein.

The eventual upshot of our discussions was that in 2012 we set up a community based organisation (CBO) in Kenya, called *Kepsteno Rotwo* ('Abandon the Knife' in Pokot language). We now have a successful working model in Pokot which given more resources could easily be replicated elsewhere.

We are having considerable success with Alternative Rite of Passage (ARP) ceremonies. Over the past five years more than 1,250 girls have participated. The *Guardian* has a film people can see of our ceremonies (*Abandon the Knife*) and we continue to forge ahead into ever more remote villages, training many traditional birth attendants (called TBAs), the majority of whom were formerly circumcisers.

We are now trying also to raise funds for training chiefs and elders who largely turn a blind eye to FGM, even though they know it's illegal. We recently held a big public event in Sigor, Central Pokot, to mark February 6th, the International Day of Zero Tolerance to FGM. The Health Minister was Guest of Honour with many chiefs and elders in attendance.

Late last year (2014) we launched a poster campaign in Central Pokot, sponsored by *The Guardian*, to reach people in remote rural areas with high prevalence of FGM who have very little access to information or media such as radio, TV or newspapers. The winning design from around three hundred submitted by local girls was printed onto huge billboards, then erected around the County.

But new challenges and perils continue to arise. One of our group members from Kepsteno Rotwo (KR) told me last year, 'Cathy, there's a new danger!'

KR members were recently invited to a remote mountainous village in Central Pokot, where a young woman (aged about 17) had died in August during childbirth. The unfortunate girl was held down by her own two brothers and forcibly cut during the pregnancy, and then cut again during delivery, when tragically she bled to death.

I have been reliably informed that this forced FGM is sometimes done as a punishment to the girl for becoming pregnant. People don't know whether the sexual intercourse was consensual or not – as if it matters during delivery – but of course the responsibility is laid at the girl's door.

Also, sometimes the TBA performs FGM at delivery because of her superstition that she cannot deliver an uncircumcised woman/girl.

We visited the village subsequently to raise awareness of the dangers of FGM and the illegality. We need to empower girls to refuse FGM and continue at school.

FGM is definitely reducing in the areas where we have worked. Robust follow up in

2012 revealed only 5 per cent of the girls who had participated in our programme had subsequently had FGM. Likewise, recent statistics in Kenya show a reduction from 27 per cent a few years ago, to 21 per cent currently.

I don't think we can afford to include male circumcision alongside FGM at this stage of the campaign, not because there are not human rights and health issues, but because the consequences are usually nowhere near as extreme as those for women and girls, especially the longer term devastating consequences such as during childbirth, dyspareunia, and the list goes on. I almost feel that male and female genital mutilation are two separate issues.

There are other important issues also to consider, in parallel with FGM.

Obstetric fistulae are common and are the indirect result of FGM, either following obstructed labour or because during the delivery traditional birth assistants cut the woman to make room for the baby to deliver, but may cut through the rectum as well. Also, early forced marriage following FGM is another indirect cause of fistula (via obstructed labour).

As a campaigner I spend large amount of my free time on fund raising (massive challenge), travelling to Pokot during annual leave at my own expense, emailing, phone calls to Kenya, organising and managing activities. We at Beyond FGM have had great fun doing sponsored coast to coast bike rides, triathlons, caving, Go-Ape and comedy nights at the local pub.

I also keep my own training up to date, and have undertaken the Level 6 FGM Training and Management course at University College Hospital in London. It is wrong that those trying both to support affected women and girls and to prevent FGM are constantly struggling for funds to carry out this much needed service and campaigning. A lot of support is provided by unpaid volunteers within communities in our cities.

First and foremost we need political will from every quarter, including the larger UN bodies. To repeat: practical action has to happen at the grassroots. Last time we asked for support was at the UN Head Quarters in Nairobi. After much hassle to secure a meeting with a senior member of UNFPA, I was told, 'Sorry we don't fund small organisations anymore.'

A recent UNICEF report from The Gambia says at the current rate of decline it will take another 125 years for the rate to fall from 76 to 30 per cent. We know what the problems are, we don't need more conferences in hallowed halls.

There is a growing global movement that sees FGM as one of the most serious human rights violations of our age. I feel it is a major feminist issue, a socialist issue.

Given all these real and urgent problems, I find it shocking and unacceptable that labiaplasty has increased massively on the NHS in the UK, whilst asylum in the UK for those who fear FGM is often not granted. I feel strongly that women and girls escaping forced FGM should be given asylum.

Also, FGM definitely has a negative economic impact, which has not really been studied in depth, but of course when a young woman or girl drops out of school she immediately suffers a potential economic loss.

Grassroots activism and education, education, education is the way forward. Get out of the ivory towers and work on the ground with communities.

This is a most urgent human rights issue of our time, the human rights of the girl child. It has profound and devastating effects at the time and for the rest of the child's life.

I beg decision makers to turn their attention to the grassroots, where change actually happens.

***

Ann-Marie Wilson

It was in 2005, when I was working for an international aid organisation in West Darfur, Sudan, that I first came across female genital mutilation.

I met an eleven-year-old girl in a refugee camp who had had FGM at the age of five. When the girl was ten her village was attacked, her family killed and she was raped. She survived the rape but was left alone and pregnant. After months of hardship the girl was found by aid workers, struggling with obstructed labour as a result of the FGM. Fortunately they were able to get her to a medical centre and thanks to the skill of the doctors and nurses, both the young mother and her baby survived.

I was so moved by this girl's story that I decided to find out more about FGM and what could be done to prevent it happening to other girls. Five years of training and research later, I had discovered the horrifying extent and implications of FGM. Learning about FGM, now some ten years ago, has meant that I have chosen to work in that field as a cause ever since.

During those first five years I also learnt that, despite the brave work of anti-FGM campaigners in some countries, there was little or no support for women who had undergone FGM and very few effective programmes to eradicate the practice and protect future generations of girls. I therefore founded *28 Too Many* in 2010, to research FGM in the 28 African countries where it is practised and to encourage and support local interventions to support those affected and accelerate the eradication of this harmful practice.

Multi agency, joined up focus across all agencies/organisations is essential to deliver both the eradication of FGM and the much-needed care those who have already undergone it require. Education and health rights must be met, and change must be fostered from within communities rather than imposing it from outside. Community engagement is critical to success.

Our research shows that FGM has reduced in some countries, but better quality data is needed to accurately assess change. As a general trend we are seeing that the more communities are aware of FGM, the more (in some cases) this results in secrecy and the practice is going underground to avoid detection and possible arrests.

The wider society has a duty to protect the vulnerable, which includes protection from FGM as an issue of human rights and child abuse. *28TooMany* also focusses on wider intimate partner violence, sexual and gender-based violence and all harmful traditional practices (often called IPVs, SGBV, and HTPs).

It is still usually very difficult for anyone to speak out against FGM from within a practising community. Those standing against FGM can face threats, social exclusion and even physical violence, especially as these are very sensitive issues and influential members of society may be resistant to change.

We therefore seek new ways to challenge FGM. For example, on the International Day of Zero Tolerance to FGM 2015 we were pleased to announce our exciting new project in Kenya. Along with our partners, the Maasai Cricket Warriors, and Cricket Without Boundaries, our project team will deliver a special programme, which uses cricket as the vehicle to work with local communities, empower young people and deliver important health and anti-FGM education.

Our work needs to be Africa-led. Survivors must have a voice, and we must work with men and boys as well as women and girls. Faith has a place in our campaigns, and faith leaders must be ready to engage and influence change. We must also focus consistently on education and awareness.

Change can happen; and it has already started.

***

Hazel Barrett

I had known about female genital mutilation for a while, but it was during a research trip to The Gambia in the late 1980s that I first became aware FGM was still being practised.

A colleague and I were researching the economic and social impacts of externally funded vegetable gardens for women, designed to improve their livelihoods and the nutrition of their families. All the projects were doing well, supplying vegetables to the local markets during the dry season when most horticultural goods had to be imported and of course prices were high.

One day my colleague and I visited the women's vegetable garden in Lamin, which had received European Union funding and had a solar powered irrigation system. This group of women were experienced in growing vegetables and had a contract to supply produce to a local trader. The quality of the produce was excellent and there were clear economic benefits to the women, their families and the village.

However, on this day we found nobody tending the crop, which had clearly not been irrigated for some days. The plants were dying and the harvest was rotting in the sun.

When we enquired what the problem was, we were told there was a big celebration in the village for girls who had had FGM. As FGM had not been performed in the village for a number of years, every family had a girl who had been cut and therefore all the women were involved in preparing food and occupied by the celebrations. We were told that because of this the women had not had time to tend their vegetable garden.

The FGM celebration clearly took priority over the project and the contract they had signed. Needless to say the trader looked elsewhere to fulfil his contract and it took many years for the Lamin Women's Vegetable Cooperative to gain the confidence of other traders and secure a reliable alternative outlet for their produce.

And tragically, there was absolutely no good reason for that disastrous 'celebration'. FGM has no health benefits. FGM has both negative physical and psychological impacts on the girls and women who have been subjected to it. FGM affects girls and women throughout their life course and impacts on their closest relationships, namely with their parents and later with their husbands.

Occasions in a woman's life which should be a time of celebration, such as marriage and having children, are tinged with FGM and the pain it brings and the mental trauma associated with it. No religion condones FGM. FGM is a form of sexual control of girls and women that impacts on their bodily integrity and human rights.

In 2015, we know that female genital mutilation is the most common cause of child abuse in the UK. When performed on adult women, it is a form of gender-based violence. It must be stopped.

Along with our REPLACE2 research programmes in other European countries, we are also working on a project in the UK, developing a web app, funded by Coventry University and the Eleanor Rathbone, Pamela Barlow and 1970 Trusts, which is designed to raise awareness of FGM amongst young people in Britain.

The web app, which can be accessed on a smart phone, tablet or laptop, contains information on FGM, the views of women and men, has a quiz and FAQs, and gives information on where young people can get help and advice on issues concerning FGM.

The app will be launched in June 2015 before the school summer holidays, which is a peak time for girls to be sent to their home countries to have the FGM performed on them.

FGM is part of my professional life. Undertaking research on such an emotive topic inevitably becomes an important part of my personal experience. I also spend much of my own time raising awareness of FGM and giving talks and presentations. I will continue to speak up against FGM and to promote a behavioural change approach to ending it, working with communities.

I am an academic, researcher and a professor in Development Geography. I believe this gives me respect both within affected communities, and with campaigners, the media and policy makers. I intend to continue with my research and am applying for funding to this end. There is much to do! I would like funding to apply the REPLACE Approach to practising communities outside the EU, perhaps in North America and Africa.

FGM has significant economic impact, in terms of cost of medical treatment, time lost to work etc, in many parts of the world. I am however more concerned with the human cost.

I first became aware of the practice of FGM whilst a student at the University of Sussex in the School of African and Asian Studies. It was during the 1970s when Women in Development had started to be topical, following the publication of Ester Boserup's seminal analysis *Woman's role in economic development* (1970, reprinted 2007). It was a time of great optimism for women and their right to benefit from the fruits of development.

I would never have predicted that, 40 years later, female genital mutilation was still being performed. It is a scandal.

....

PROFESSIONALS IN WIDER ROLES

CLINICIANS

Phoebe Abe-Okwonga was born in Uganda and is now a medical general practitioner in the UK. She offers here expert perspectives and advice on the treatment of women and girls in Britain who have undergone female genital mutilation. Phoebe attended Medical School at Makerere University in Uganda, but in 1971-79 had to flee to the UK as a refugee from the brutal Idi Amin led administration in that country. She completed her Medical School studies in the UK and also obtained a Master's degree in Tropical Diseases. She is an associate member on the UK Parliament APPG *(All Parliamentary Party Group)* on FGM and provides free clinics at her practice for survivors of FGM.

Dr J. is a medical general practitioner in Scotland. She has extensive family planning and obstetric experience and reports a growing awareness amongst her colleagues of the possibility that patients who present for treatment may have undergone FGM. She alerts us to the wider challenges of providing quality individual health care for patients with this condition, whilst Dr F, a Public Health consultant with particular responsibility for FGM matters in a local authority (council) in the

North West of England, provides a public health perspective.

***

Phoebe Abe-Okwonga

I grew up in Uganda, but whilst still a medical student there I had to seek refuge in the UK, to escape the perils of Idi Amin's brutal hold at that time on my country. Then, in 1983, I lost my husband, a consultant surgeon, who died in an unexplained helicopter crash in Uganda. I therefore had to bring up five children on my own, which had guided me to a special concern for widows and other single mothers in my country of birth.

I continue to visit Uganda when I can and whilst visiting Northern Uganda to work with the Acholi women and young people, I have managed to buy few acres where they can do small farming. Millet, cassava, beans, groundnuts, and maize have given some yields, which are sold to pay children's school fees, and the women also do some subsistence farming, rearing pigs and chicken and growing vegetables, fruits, and plantain on this small plot of land.

I am now a medical general practitioner in the UK and, over the years, I have also found myself supporting many women and girls here, especially those who have had FGM. My general practice is in Hillingdon, North London, and slowly word has got out that I seek to help these women.

I run a daily clinic, free of charge, in my practice for any woman or girl who needs advice about how to cope with the problems FGM brings. The clinic also offers group meetings and informal companionship with other women who have experienced this affliction.

Two such groups are the 100 Black Women in the UK is group of Afro-Caribbean British Women in the diaspora who are working together to empower one another, and FAW (Female Genital Mutilation Association Worldwide), a group was set up in 2013, inspired by FGM survivors attending my GP clinics in Berkshire and Middlesex, and so-named by them.

Working to support FGM survivors in Britain is another aspect of the same campaign for human dignity and well-being. My work here has mainly focussed on ethnic minorities, talking and singing to and with them in different schools around England, and, increasingly, at national conferences, where I've shared my experience of the problems FGM brings.

My focus on the arts as well as medicine has enabled me to support a wide range of people in exploring positive ways to shape their futures, whilst also raising money through sales for charitable work.

Members of FAW (the newly formed FGM Association Worldwide, of which Valentine Nkoyo is President) meet with me regularly in our surgery or in our homes. We also attend and organise conferences.

An important aspect of my UK medical work is the daily free and open-access clinics at my Berkshire and Middlesex practices, which I set up for women with FGM. Current attendance is about 70 patients, of whom more than a dozen are younger than 15. Their problems are complex, and often complicated by cultural contexts and family situations.

For example, I have three patients currently waiting to be seen for de-infibulation, but in each case their spouse is still resisting or refusing to support them:

- Mrs A's spouse lives in Somalia and she goes there to visit him. She wants to fall pregnant and but has secondary infertility simply because she is so tight at the vaginal entrance, which is approximately 1cm diameter. She already has one child aged seven who is disabled because of a very difficult labour; she was eventually delivered by emergency Caesarean section.

- Mrs B's spouse lives in Sudan. They are separated but he still insists that she must not receive the repair. Mrs B has many medical problems and a ten-year-old child, also delivered by emergency Caesarean section.

- Mrs C is divorced from her ex-spouse. Both live in the UK. He is telling her not to be de-infibulated although she has so far required two elective Caesarean sections. I am trying to convince her to get help because she has so many medical complications.

The service I provide is a non-funded GP booked clinic for ten or twenty minute appointment from Mondays to Fridays at the Yiewsley Family Practice for any females (and their families) wanting to discuss medical, social or psychological issues pertaining to FGM.

As a general practitioner (GP) I am able to physically examine (with or without the presence of a nurse assistant), investigate, treat, manage and if necessary refer to any specific specialties as necessary, free within the NHS system. This offers the patient proper care in all areas of our medical setting. I am not just treating FGM, but looking after a person.

I attend to diagnosis, coding, and the management of specific stages of FGM, especially Type III.

Long term care after deinfibulation is imperative. This can also have slight or rare complications and problems, and patients are counselled and advised before and after their minor operations. Sometimes over the years they might have developed adhesions, scaring and keloids and (rarely) fistulae, but more commonly they have chronic urine incontinence and problems needing special care and follow through with a continuing community doctor-patient relationship.

There are numerous medical and health complications that come with FGM. There are acute and chronic problems; I usually see the latter cases, as most patients arrive having had FGM years earlier.

Also, child safeguarding is important. Most of these women have young children and may not have their fathers around. I am fortunate to be a member of the Hillingdon Child Safeguarding Committee, where we meet regularly to discuss issues regarding all safety to children in the borough and if necessary I bring attention to FGM issues.

The role of men in combating FGM is crucial. This is part of the message on that theme which I shared at a Fringe Meeting at the Labour Party Conference in 2014:

> *The men are the head of the household in our African community. As such we need them to start talking to one another, with real dialogue and discussion ...*
>
> *Let us make sure that no more girls will suffer from the pain of 'cutting'. They are our children. They are your children. No one loves girls more than their fathers. The bond and love between daughters and fathers is like honey and bees.*
>
> *I therefore call upon men and women all over the world to support and empower the FGM women survivors, the girls and their brothers. This will make them strong and healthy to support their men, their family and the nations. A healthy and happy woman is a healthy family. The old English adage is, 'Behind every successful man there is a strong woman'. Let's have a new African saying: 'Next to every man standing there is a strong woman'.*

✳✳✳

Dr J

Female genital mutilation is universally recognised by clinicians as a potential cause of physical and mental ill-health, but the indirect risks go even further than that. To be effective, even routine health care can demand a different or more nuanced approach.

One example is a patient, a childless woman recently arrived from sub-Saharan Africa, who had been asked to attend my general practice for a routine cervical smear (pap) test. It had taken several efforts to persuade her to attend at all, but when she came I couldn't get the speculum in to see her cervix because the introitus (vagina) was very tightly sewn and it was painful for her.

The lady said she had been cut years ago at home. This continues to be the case for some patients. It is known that FGM in Scotland is a hidden phenomenon, frequently undetected – which means women who have FGM may be reluctant to seek medical help for that or any other condition, or even to take their 'cut' daughters for any medical care, for fear of legal or other consequences.

I referred this patient to a gynaecologist, as she told me she was consistently suffering from painful sex and also wanted children. It was important thereafter to support her to keep her hospital appointments. There is increased risk with FGM that even conceiving and, if a pregnancy occurs, subsequent delivery, will present problems.

We must bear in mind too that support with family planning – very important for the well-being of women and their families everywhere – is also quite challenging in some situations where the patient has had FGM. This is particularly so, for example, for IUD or IUS (coil) insertion, which are good methods for women who require a discreet way to limit family size, whatever their husbands' preferences.

There can also be difficult issues around the health care of women who seek asylum on the grounds of possible FGM or forced marriage, for themselves or their daughters.

Further, if a woman who has FGM then gives birth to a daughter, there is a possibility (by no means certainty) that the child will likewise be subjected to FGM. The health visitor must without exception be informed proactively, so any risk to the little girl can be assessed and, if necessary, dealt with, before she comes to harm.

Questions about FGM status and intentions must be routine aspects of women's and children's care. Doctors and nurse practitioners must be trained in this, and be consistently aware of the possible risks.

Some (not all, of course) patients from diaspora communities have little understanding of how their bodies work, why they should have routine precautionary health care, or why FGM is dangerous child abuse. The mother (or father) may be opposed to FGM, but the other parent or another family member could still try to engineer it. The risks of harm are sometimes real, whatever the main caregiver's stated position.

Even whether patients will attend for normal procedures such as smear tests or breast examinations can be in question, if a woman has had FGM. There could also be issues for her (and her husband, who perhaps wants to control what she does), when it comes to modesty and physical examinations.

There are other non-gynaecological physical and psychological problems that may, for reasons of access, modesty or lack of information, also remain unaddressed. We need to think about the whole person when we try to provide health care, especially for marginalised patients.

It's encouraging to see FGM being brought to public attention in Scotland; for people to be helped, we need to get the topic out in the open. Recently there was a play about FGM at the Traverse Theatre in Edinburgh, and that will help encourage people to think more freely about this illegal and serious threat to the health and well-being of women and their families.

*****

Dr F

It was about 1999 when I read a book in which a story about female genital mutilation was told through the eyes of a victim. That was when I first became aware of FGM, what it was, and how it affected people's lives. Then from about 2001, as a specialist in public health, I became more aware of FGM in the context of the sexual health agenda. I am even more aware of this issue now that I work on the children' and violence prevention agendas.

I have not witnessed FGM directly, but am aware of the potential scale of the problem through reading published documents and reports. (I say 'potential' scale simply because FGM is still hidden within communities.)

We ensure in my local health authority that there are policies in place to pick up FGM cases, in particular within maternity and sexual health services. We are of the understanding that there is (fortunately) very little FGM here within our communities. However, we do discuss the FGM policy at our Local Safeguarding Children Board and we do work with the police and health professionals to be assured that if FGM were to take place, the relevant persons (officers and other professionals) would be informed and support provided for the individual.

It's important that mainstream services are active in stopping FGM – it's about reducing harm in our community and what we can do to support different communities. If we only approach issues on a 'community by community basis' we are less likely to bring about change.

We must recognise the emotional, physical and long-term impacts of FGM, and the fact that usually these are children when it happens (although, please note, it shouldn't happen at any age). The reasons why it happens – based on cultural beliefs, which are not really understood – must also be acknowledged. The context of FGM is usually within the community, happening to young girls.

Working together within communities; raising the awareness; and advocating for change so that this 'practice' is not carried out any more are all essential to eradication. We must keep the discussions going.

....

EDUCATION AND PUBLIC SERVICES

Schools and other public services are obviously central in work to ensure girls do not experience the child abuse of female genital mutilation. Here a girls' school head-teacher and the chair of the Local Safeguarding Children Board (LSCB) in Islington, London, explain their roles in child safeguarding against FGM.

Gladys Berry is head teacher of a multicultural girls' school in North London. Gladys and her colleagues have been collaborating with the school's local authority, Islington, in the innovative development of age-appropriate curriculum to address the risks and, sometimes, reality of female genital mutilation, for the girls in her care.

Alan Caton OBE is the Independent Chair for the Local Safeguarding Children Boards in Islington and Central Bedfordshire. He was previously a police officer in Suffolk Constabulary and from 2008 the head of Suffolk Constabulary's Public Protection Directorate.

Gladys Berry

As the Head of a large multicultural girls' school in Islington, London, I have been aware of FGM for a long time. A white, ethnic Irish professional, I have taught for 33 years and been a head teacher for six years. I have taught science in inner city multicultural schools for most of my career. I have had quite a lot of experience teaching the biology of sex, but also in creating sensitive learning environments within which children and young people can feel confident about asking questions concerning HIV, sexuality, gender and related topics.

Students in our school now have lessons on FGM. One of our students has been Youth Mayor for Islington for the last two years and has run her own campaign against FGM. She was interviewed by the television channel ITN. It is good to see campaigning on female genital mutilation, and for there to be a level of media attention to it. It is finally in the minds of a significant number of people.

Our school has very close links with other agencies, including Social Services, Families First and The Child and Adolescent Mental Health Service (*CAMHS*). We buy in additional CAMHS hours. We also have a school-based Safer Schools Police Officer who is very approachable. Our local authority have been very good at signposting support for FGM work in school and they promoted the development of lesson materials which we trialled for them.

As a school we have invested in our Inclusion team and are very effective in creating an environment within which students feel safe to tell us things. So far, we have experience from the Somali community. In the past this community has felt hard to reach. We now have a Somali Science and Maths club facilitated by a worker from the Somali Centre.

We contribute to some of the costs of this, but the Somali Centre contributes most of the resource. This provision means our early stage English learners have additional support. It also acts as a club that promotes and values the education of girls and helps us engage with parents, not just through translation. Feedback from students after they have had these lessons shows that students would be more willing to speak out having had the lessons. Acquisition of the English language by early stage English language students is a barrier to begin with.

We are uncertain about the extent of this issue within our school community. It does affect my everyday life, because we know we have a small number of students who have had this done, and we also suspect there may be more who have not disclosed to us. We also have parents who are worried and do not want it to happen to their daughters.

This must be addressed by wider society, absolutely. It must not be allowed to become or remain a matter within any enclave. It also must not be allowed to become a focus for racist attitudes towards any part of the community.

This is another important example of how girls and women are considered in terms of being sexual objects without will, reason or purpose. There is a lot of work that needs to be done to make our society a better and healthier place for girls and young women from all parts of the community. Talking about FGM needs to be normalised.

There are still related issues that need to be discussed, for instance questions about male circumcision or female genital cosmetic surgery. Essentially, I disagree with any medical intervention being carried out unnecessarily, if not in the best interests of the child's health and well-being. With respect to FGM reconstructive surgery I think the woman should be given enough information and understanding to decide for herself if this is something that will be beneficial for her.

I do think however there should be more prosecutions of medical and other workers, in this country, who have engaged in FGM procedures.

There has been politically correct lip service paid to this at national level, as if it is a fashionable thing to have a conscience about. We must make FGM political.

Get FGM on to the national agenda. It is not there yet because, when the topic is FGM, we are talking about little girls, and they are not deemed sufficiently important.

***

Alan Caton

As head of Suffolk Constabulary's Public Protection Directorate from 2008 to 2013, I took the lead on child protection, domestic abuse, prostitution and sexual exploitation, forced marriage and female genital mutilation. It was in this role that I first heard from victims of this barbaric act.

I was aware of FGM in the early 2000s, and that laws existed which banned the act of FGM, but at that time I knew very little about the issue. There is no doubt, however, that FGM, identifying victims of it and prosecuting offenders, is now becoming a priority for many agencies.

In 2013 I retired from the police force and became the Independent Chair for two Local Safeguarding Children Boards (LSCBs), in Islington and Central Bedfordshire. Recent government guidance (Working Together to Safeguard Children 2015) makes it clear that LSCBs should agree with local authorities and partners about the levels and different types of assessment and services to be commissioned and delivered. This includes, amongst other things, children who have undergone or may undergo female genital mutilation.

I view FGM as a horrific act of child abuse. Within my LSCB's influence, partner agencies to do all they can to identify and support victims of FGM and to bring perpetrators to account for carrying out acts of FGM.

I would like to think that most local authority children's social care, health professionals and the police are becoming well informed about this issue and that in most authorities there will be practitioners experienced in FGM-related child protection issues and therefore have professionals available to support and assist those in need.

Other harmful traditional practices that LSCB's should be focussing on include, honour based abuse, early child and forced marriage, abuse linked to a belief in spirit possession and breast-ironing also known as breast-flattening.

Politicians also need to raise the issue of FGM on the world stage, and nationally there must be greater awareness of the issue and the extreme harm it causes to children and young women.

There needs to be an overarching strategy that requires all agencies to understand the issues of FGM. There is not one agency that can deal with this matter alone, but collectively the power of all agencies working together can be immense and deliver successful outcomes. For example, effective referral paths, police and other agency intelligence and prioritising the issues across the board are all critical.

It is very difficult for those communities affected to speak out, mainly through fear. Safeguarding is everyone's responsibility and we must ensure that everyone knows what action to take if they have concerns about a child – namely call the police or children's social care. Or, if there are issues with reporting to the authorities, use an 'FGM Helpline' which concerned people can call for advice and support.

Whilst there is already legislation within the UK to combat this issue, the fact that there have been no successful prosecutions makes it very clear that we must take a different approach.

Eradicating female genital mutilation must be a government priority. This is a most barbaric, cruel and violent practice that impacts on children and women for the whole of their lives.

....

LEGAL AND HUMAN RIGHTS

Female genital mutilation is a very complex matter, not least in its legal aspects. Here four campaigners with direct experience of the law and of supporting FGM survivors consider some of these issues, such as legislation, asylum claims and how the police perceive matters.

Karl Turner is a Member of Parliament and a barrister (attorney) who is currently Shadow Solicitor General, a remit which includes human rights and the Crown Prosecution Service.

Dexter Dias QC is a London-based human rights barrister (Queen's Counsel) and a part-time Crown Court judge. He is also a researcher at Cambridge and Harvard Universities.

Anj Handa lives in Leeds, UK, and is co-director of People Help People Ltd, a consultancy which tithes a percentage of commercial profits across to the People Help People Foundation, which addresses issues such as women and girls and human rights, including asylum seekers.

Mr K has professional experience of working in the British legal system. He considers particularly the complex relationships between FGM and female genital cosmetic surgery, also known as FGCS.

Karl Turner

I am a Labour member of parliament and Shadow Solicitor General, which means I am Labour's spokesperson in the House of Commons on issues such as the Crown Prosecution Service and human rights.

Prior to being an MP, I was a practising barrister in Chambers in Hull, in the northeast of England. I saw on a daily basis the effect that government policy can have on communities. I am, therefore, confident that changes in approach to female genital mutilation in this Parliament can over the next few years have positive effect and bring about real change.

The fight against FGM isn't a recent phenomenon. Campaigns have been run to combat the practice over several decades. My own party, Labour, has plenty of dedicated individuals who want to ensure the plight of thousands of young girls and women does not go unnoticed, and that individuals and groups carrying out this act will be brought to justice under the full weight of the law.

As an MP, it is my responsibility to keep the issue of FGM in the government's minds and in the spotlight of public consciousness. I continue to do this in many ways.

I am a member of the All-Party Parliamentary Group (APPG) on Female Genital Mutilation, and I have held debates in the House of Commons and tabled parliamentary questions, as well as asking my fellow MPs to join me in the fight against this deplorable act. I have met with special prosecutors from a number of countries who are able to demonstrate clear and effective ways of ensuring that FGM is tackled. This practical approach enables me to raise the issues and keep the pressure on.

Combating FGM requires concerted efforts to bridge the gap between law and social policy. Much of the legislation that we pass in parliament has the best intention, but it is toothless unless it is backed up in a practical way. There needs to be a joined up approach, tackling FGM in both the public and private spheres.

So what does a joined up approach look like? Firstly we need to ensure that those in relevant public roles are sufficiently trained to deal with this very sensitive issue. The police, nurses, doctors, teachers, social workers and others must all know how to spot the signs of FGM and how best to deal with any situations that may arise.

Secondly, the personnel of organisations dealing specifically with FGM should be drawn from a wide variety of backgrounds, to facilitate insights into the complex and sensitive cultural issues that surround the practice. We cannot expect improved outcomes in the fight against FGM if our police force is predominantly white male; and this applies to other institutions also. We must push for a more diverse public sector overall, to meet the needs and challenges that FGM and other traditional harmful practices (such as forced and 'early' marriage – child rape – and child grooming) present.

Thirdly, criminals who carry out the act of FGM must be prosecuted and brought to justice. The UK lags woefully behind other countries when it comes to the arrest and prosecution of those who carry out this act. It is a shocking statistic that, even though up to fifty British girls and women a day, perhaps more, are at risk of FGM, there has never been a single successful prosecution in the UK.

FGM, like other crimes against women, is notoriously difficult to prosecute. Often involving young girls who go through extreme trauma and pain, the practice occurs in private and often times in other countries. Appointing and training specialist officers and prosecutors who can spot the signs of FGM will mean investigations and prosecutions will be carried out in a sensitive but thorough way. Mandatory reporting of concerns about abuse by professionals in regulated activity (such as teachers and nurses) is also required.

Lastly, we must include a wide spectrum of civil society organisations, as well as survivors of this barbaric act, in policy making. By increasing the number of potential stakeholders in government policy we support communities to take control of their own complex and sensitive cultural issues, and are able more effectively to tackle this persistent problem.

We must also ensure that schools and local authorities take the problem of FGM seriously and put in place measures to make it easier to spot and report. Education is vital if FGM is to be eradicated. When young people know that what they may experience or hear is wrong, that will make it easier to track down those who carry out this criminal act.

As a legislator, it is my job to ensure that laws in the best interest of the wider public are passed. Whilst the previous, Coalition Government passed legislation that made it easier to tackle FGM, there are still important steps to take. Labour has put forward coherent plans to tackle FGM and we hope we shall gain cross-party support.

Yvette Cooper, when she was Shadow Home Secretary, went on record as calling for FGM protection orders to be put in place, to make it more difficult to take children abroad for 'vacation cutting', and we want civil courts to be given legal powers to intervene.

The campaign against FGM in Parliament has come on leaps and bounds, especially in the 2010–2015 Parliament, but there is still a long way to go. The Home Affairs Select Committee recently released a scathing report into the practice stating that:

> FGM is an ongoing national scandal, which is likely to have resulted in the preventable mutilation of thousands of girls. Successive governments, politicians, the police, health, education and social care sectors should all share responsibility for the failure to respond adequately to the growing prevalence of FGM in the UK.

Whilst there are legislators like myself and others to keep FGM on the agenda, we have a good chance of eradicating this practice from British shores. We want to establish an example to follow, for other countries around the globe that must also confront this horrendous human rights abuse.

***

Dexter Dias

It was a no-brainer for me as a human rights lawyer. FGM is one of the most egregious violations of human rights in the world and, what is more, it is inflicted on some of the most vulnerable people, in their millions, every year.

My legal chambers in London were created to represent those disadvantaged by different forms of poverty and discrimination. A significant part of my legal and research work contests gender-based violence, of which FGM is one of the severest manifestations.

Although the UK criminalised FGM in the 1980s, infamously there were no prosecutions in almost three decades. Beyond this stark fact, it was increasingly clear to those of us working in human rights law that the UK's overall institutional response and protective mechanisms were seriously defective.

I have worked and campaigned with survivors for a number of years, and we sought to forge strategic, innovative alliances to exert power on the organs of state to strengthen their response to FGM. This culminated in the announcement in 2013 that there would be a Parliamentary Inquiry into FGM.

I was determined that our national scrutiny of the practice should be strongly imbued with human rights sensibility. As such I argued for, and succeeded in securing, the creation of a working group of the Bar Human Rights Committee (BHRC) to respond to the Parliamentary Inquiry. Our stance was to critique the UK's response to FGM, meticulously evaluating this response against the nation's international treaty obligations, not only in regard to FGM, but also in regard to the vindication of the rights of women and children.

We concluded that the UK has been in breach of its international law obligations to protect young women and girls from mutilation.

During the period of the UK's breach of its obligations, thousands of British girls and young women have been unnecessarily exposed to the risk of mutilation and have suffered irreparable physical and emotional damage. Many could – and should – have been saved. This constituted a serious breach of the state's duty of care. Immediate remedial action had to be taken. To this end, the BHRC made twelve recommendations for urgent implementation.

Our proposals were broadly endorsed by Parliament. In particular, the government adopted our recommendation that a new legal tool was required to enhance the protective mechanism: FGM Protection Orders.

These Orders are now the law of the land and are being used by the High Court to proactively intervene to protect girls from mutilation. A step in the right direction. There is still a long way to go.

***

Anj Handa

Waris Dirie's book, *Desert Flower*, which I read now around twenty years ago, was the text that initially alerted me to the facts of female genital mutilation. At the time, I didn't know what I could do about it. I was a recent graduate working in the corporate sector, but it clearly stuck with me.

Moving forward, I'm now a director of People Help People, a social business which includes the People Help People Foundation, so that we can tithe our own profits or time into supporting End FGM. I began to campaign about FGM in late 2013, mostly tweeting and sharing articles by Hilary Burrage and other prominent End FGM campaigners.

Then, in January 2014, I was introduced to an FGM survivor, Afusat Saliu, and began work to support her with her asylum case. Through this work I also learnt a lot on a personal level about what it is like to live with FGM, both psychologically and physically/sexually.

I'm not sure whether the incidence of FGM is decreasing, but I know a Leeds-based organisation, Gambia Volunteers, has been undertaking a significant amount of work on educating men in their communities, here in the UK and in Gambia.

This is the reason Dr Jean Garrod (my business partner) and I produced the FGM in Leeds report, on a *pro bono* basis. We knew that the charities and grassroots organisations didn't have the evidence base relating to the scale and were often being fobbed off by funding bodies locally and nationally. We have both found our research / policy / strategy background useful, as this is something the smaller organisations tend to lack and we are able to support them in this area.

Although we are not a grassroots organisation, we support these groups with small pieces of pro bono work. We also attend their events, such as the Bradford FGM conference and fundraising dinner in March led by Peacemaker International, where Jean and I were presented with an award for our work.

I continue to tweet, blog and share articles on Facebook about FGM. My particular area of concern is FGM in the context of asylum. It's a largely overlooked area. I feel it often goes hand in hand with forced marriage.

As a campaigner, many people will wish you to stop putting your head above the parapet. FGM is an uncomfortable subject for many and you may find yourself losing friends – but I will always prefer friends who stand for something. There may be trolls, and there may be those who can't understand why you're doing this.

Your wellbeing as a campaigner is important – give yourself time for self-care.

I'd like the decision makers to stop pouring most of the money into expensive marketing campaigns such as Girl Generation, and instead support the grassroots organisations that need resources and can make a difference.

Regarding more down to earth aspects of debates around FGM, I'd think that male circumcision (MGM) is a topic which people might also consider alongside FGM, but I haven't focussed on this area so don't have much to contribute. I am however sure that FGM has significant economic impact.

Some of the physical problems of FGM survivors are usually addressed (for those that actually present for healthcare services), but it's the back pains, depression and do forth that can often prevent women from holding down a job. We need much better psychological care and understanding for survivors.

***

Mr K

The fight to eradicate FGM requires both that the criminal justice system works in conjunction with the education, health and social services and the third sector (NGOs), and that, through engagement, there is a willingness in the practising communities to eradicate this custom. A number of unresolved questions around the status of female genital cosmetic surgery make this objective more difficult.

Some of the main issues to address regarding FGM within the African community include:

- training front line professionals on awareness of the practice,
- better referrals of FGM incidents to the police from other frontline agencies,
- a Statutory Mandatory Reporting Law to protect children at risk,
- addressing the issue of female genital cosmetic surgery (FGCS) and
- co-operation from the affected community.

Most frontline services have now introduced measures to train staff on how to identify FGM; for instance, FGM is now mandated as part of personal development training in the Metropolitan Police. The NHS and education services are also beginning to make progress with training and awareness.

The government has recently introduced routine recording of all FGM victims/cases in hospitals and in Primary Care Trusts, and the *Serious Crime Bill* 2015 contains measures to allow examination of children at risk of FGM, so progress has also commenced on that front.

The Government has consulted on introducing a mandatory reporting regulation for FGM in England and Wales. This contentious regulation will require only confirmed cases in children (under 18-year-old girls) to be reported mandatorily.

The issue of female genital cosmetic surgery (FGCS) is therefore the only issue listed above that is not being actively looked into. The Government has largely failed to consider formally the application of the current legislation in relation to FGCS. This quandary has been described as follows:

> *FGM and female genital cosmetic surgery may involve partial excision of external female genital tissue for cultural reasons. Both are based on cultural expectations of how female genitalia ought to look. Similarly, FGCS can be chosen for reasons of aesthetics, the transcendence of shame and a desire to conform to a certain cultural ideal — and yet, female genital mutilation is ethically condemned and banned in many countries, including the UK, while FGCS is unregulated. Michaela et al (2012:205)*

The paper did however make a distinction, saying informed consent is present in cosmetic surgery and, at least in the case of under 18s, is necessarily absent in FGM.

The government has disregarded the Home Affairs Select Committee's recommendation for a consideration to what it called a 'presumed double standard' in the application of the law.

The Association of Chief Police Officers (ACPO) and the corporate position of the Metropolitan Police Service (MPS) is that there is a perceived double standard in which focus on FGM is placed on black and ethnic minority communities, with a different set of standards for the wider community to do FGSC in a flourishing private medical industry.

The government is failing in its duty to legislate a clear distinction between the two practices.

Instead of interpreting the spirit of parliament in passing the *2003 Act*, i.e. whether the current law includes FGCS for non-therapeutic needs, the government has shifted the burden to the judiciary. In 2014 the Home Department position was that, 'Ultimately, it would be for a court to decide if purely cosmetic surgery constitutes mutilation and is therefore illegal.'

Legitimacy and trust in the criminal justice system will be undermined if this issue is not addressed. The debate about procedural justice and its relationship with police legitimacy, trust and community co-operation has placed ACPOs and the MPs in contradictory positions in respect of the current legislation. The fact that those performing FGCS are overlooked, and the actors of FGM are persecuted, undermines due process.

Can you secure the interest of the affected community, expecting them to report those in their midst that offend against this statue, when nonetheless society at large are seemingly allowed to offend against the same law? Will they be willing to come forward if they see through this alleged double standard?

I have spoken to a few survivors of FGM who share these concerns.

There are frontline professionals who even in 2014 did not know what FGM stood for, and research has identified that two-thirds of clinical psychologists received no training in counselling victims of FGM. Those who are trained acquired their knowledge through personal development.

Nonetheless, some people have challenged the general indifference in attitude towards FGM in the UK.

Leyla Hussein, an anti-FGM activist driven to measure public perception towards FGM, made a documentary film in the Northampton area, where she conducted a petition pretending to be pro-FGM. In half an hour she secured 19 petitions from the public in support of FGM as a cultural practice in the UK.

Although her work would not be considered as a credible snapshot of public opinion, it perhaps highlights the question of cultural sensitivity, even if that 'sensitivity' may in some cases have resulted only from a fear of being thought rude or racist if one refused to sign a petition when asked by an earnest young woman with brown skin. Cultural sensitivity has long compounded the campaign to tackle FGM.

Enlightenment and better integration of our communities may enhance understanding of the acceptable norms of the general population.

. . . .

CIVIL SOCIETY AND TRADE UNIONS

Formal, legal perspectives on female genital mutilation are of small consequence if there is not also a common concern amongst professionals and other workers who have direct contact with survivors and those who may be at risk.

Carolyn Simpson is a British trade union official and feminist working in London. She is also Chair of the Southern and Eastern Region Women's Rights Committee, which has highlighted issues around female genital mutilation.

I suppose I have been aware of female genital mutilation as a phenomenon for years, but I've only relatively recently become involved in the campaign(s) to eradicate it, after I read more and heard programmes about it on BBC Radio 4. Thankfully, I've not been subjected to FGM personally, but the women and girls who have undergone it are my sisters, and their pain is my pain.

As the Chair of the (English) Southern and Eastern Region of the Trades Union Congress (SERTUC) *Women's Rights Committee*, and as an Equalities Officer for Unite (the trade union) I have been instrumental in raising awareness across the Regions of both the TUC and Unite.

We have had Hilary Burrage as a speaker at an open meeting at the TUC where FGM was the only agenda item and I continue to work with Hilary in involving as many people as I can in the eradication of this disgusting practice. I hope that, at our forthcoming AGM, the *Women's Rights Committee* will continue to have FGM as one of our work plans/actions for the year going forward.

Trade unions and the TUC itself carry out vital FGM awareness raising work and we should continue to do so wherever possible.

Some people have asked whether dealing with FGM should be left to the communities directly affected, but of course mainstream society must be active in stopping FGM. If society didn't act then we'd still be sending children up chimneys, wouldn't we?? Or preventing women from voting? Or stopping working class people from attending school? Or preventing women from becoming priests? Or preventing same sex marriage?? What a daft question ...

There have also been suggestions that male circumcision and FGM are the same issue. I don't think they are. The removal of a man or boy's foreskin is absolutely incomparable to the removal of a woman or girl's labia or clitoris and stitching up her vagina. Male circumcision can be for medical or developmental reasons, but FGM is a cruel infliction of power and torture on an individual with far reaching consequences – both medical and mental.

Intervention and prosecution in cases of FGM *must* happen. Teachers and carers must feel comfortable to report suspicions without fear of reprisals. Police, health care professionals and social care workers *must* act to help prosecutions, and people (including children) *must* be educated and brought to recognise that FGM is totally inappropriate and that such repressions are unacceptable in the 21st century regardless of race, religion or societal habits.

Politicians should take some responsibility and speak out. Bringing FGM into the open can only help in its eradication. There is no shame in talking about this and there is no racism in speaking about it either. The media should also take some responsibility in writing about FGM and getting it onto the public agenda.

....

MEDIA AND THE ARTS

The five campaigners against female genital mutilation featured here all used the written word to reach a wider public as journalists, novelists and bloggers, as well as creating reports and petitions on FGM. Maggie O'Kane is an internationally distinguished journalist, currently multimedia (investigations) editor at *The Guardian* newspaper in London. A former *Guardian* foreign correspondent, she has covered most of the world's major conflicts over the last decade. Her awards include British Journalist of the Year and Foreign Correspondent of the Year. She now leads the Guardian Global Media #EndFGM campaign – the most ambitious programme ever using global social media to combat FGM - which has recently been recognised by the accolade '*2015 British Media Awards Editorial Campaign of the Year*'.

Lizzie Presser was born in the USA and now lives and works as a journalist and researcher in Cambridge, UK. She has previously worked for the Half the Sky Movement, a multi-media project addressing the oppression of women.

Ms D is a UK citizen who spent time as a teenager in The Gambia. She now works in London as a professional with special regard to child protection issues, and is writing a novel for young people that challenges Eurocentric myths about FGM. She offers some interesting thoughts, too, on male 'circumcision' or 'MGM'.

Amanda Epe is also a British born author and EndFGM campaigner, of Nigerian heritage, who campaigns in London against FGM under the blog *MsRoseBlossom*.

Alex Buzzard is the *nom de plum* of Ralph Tilby, a UK-based management consultant who has worked with the (London) Metropolitan Police. As Tilby he submitted evidence to the 2014 Home Affairs (Vaz) Select Committee Inquiry into FGM. He has also published a novel, *Consciencia*, on the theme of FGM, in his name as a writer. Alex's judgement is that the police continue to pay greater attention to acquisitive crime than to people, at the expense of protecting the most vulnerable from violence and abuse.

***

Maggie O'Kane

In late 2013 we decided to start a *Guardian* media campaign to end female genital mutilation, beginning with the UK. We didn't know how prevalent FGM is in Britain, but there was certainly a problem to be tackled, and I believed that using social media – a technique denied earlier campaigners – would amplify the #EndFGM message in new and more effective ways.

This decision marked a very significant development for me; I see FGM as one of the most critical global issues we must face in terms of women's and children's rights.

We pulled together a very small team – initially just me and my *Guardian* colleague Mary Carson, with Hilary Burrage as our consultant, and later also with a small number of other *Guardian* staff members - and began with a change.org e-petition in early 2014, to persuade the then Secretary for Education Michael Gove MP to include FGM in the curriculum of all English schools. A schoolgirl, Fahma Mohamed, was chosen to head up the campaign, and we used social media to promote it. The change.org petition became the fastest growing campaign ever. In just a few weeks, we had a quarter of a million signatures – enough to secure a meeting between Fahma and Mr Gove and a subsequent promise from him to write to all English head teachers as we asked.

One of our US readers, Jaha Dukureh – herself a survivor of FGM – read about this campaign and started her own change.org petition, this time to ask President Obama to initiate a survey in America of the prevalence of FGM and create an action plan to halt so-called 'vacation cutting', where girls are taken from the USA to undergo FGM. This e-petition was picked up by us via daily social media searches and before long Jaha had aligned her campaign with ours.

The USA prevalence survey is now being undertaken and Jaha has become a key player in *The Guardian* campaign, which we next took to New York, with a launch awareness-raising event attended by the General Secretary of the United Nations, Ban Ki-moon and Alan Rusbridger, then Editor-in-Chief of *The Guardian*.

From New York, we moved on in later 2014 to Kenya and a meeting of the heads of all Kenya's leading media organisation at the UN headquarters in Nairobi, where Ban Ki-moon, joined by Jaha and a young Kenyan activist, Domtila Chesang, announced five international FGM grants (co-funded by the UNFPA and *The Guardian*) for key journalists to report on FGM and efforts to eradicate it in Kenya.

We also announced a Kenyan schools poster campaign to EndFGM, and an annual award, named after the veteran EndFGM campaigner Efua Dorkenoo (who died in 2014), for an African journalist who demonstrates commitment and dedication in seeking to end FGM, the prize being a two month internship *at The Guardian*'s head office in London.

Our intention is to nurture a new template, focussing especially on young people, in reporting FGM, which can be used across Africa.

Next, at the end of 2014, Jaha took the campaign to her home country, The Gambia, where with support from The Girl Generation and *The Guardian*, we hosted the first-ever (and widely reported) youth summit and trained 65 Gambian journalists – and secured a promise of land from the Gambian government for a rescue centre for those under threat of FGM.

And then, in 2015, we continued awareness-raising with another UN-related event in New York and have reported on FGM in places where the practice is barely acknowledged, such as Iran and Iraq.

In September 2015, collaborating with *change.org*, we will launch several week-long training camp academies for 165 young activists and journalists in Kenya, Nigeria and Somalia, as well as a national 'campaign truck' radio road shows in Kenya – again, models for action which we hope will become a template for future campaigns.

We work alongside all the lead editors in other areas of Guardian content to produce an inclusive programme. In 2016 we will take the Guardian #EndFGM Global Media Campaign forward to premiering a feature-length documentary with Jaha Dukureh at *Sundance* (an annual independent film festival in Utah) in January, and in June, with the Johannesburg Film Festival, premiering simultaneous TV transmissions across twenty FGM- practising African countries and via all global *Guardian* outlets.

Our aim is to employ every possible social media avenue to promote the eradication of FGM within a decade. We started with an online petition, Twitter, Facebook and Google Alerts and have since added global live-streaming facilities such as Periscope.

With social media and high level support we can reach many, many times more people than has ever before been possible. By engaging the wisdom of seasoned campaigners and the enthusiasm of committed young people, we can at last make FGM history forever.

***

Lizzie Presser

As an American, I first became aware of female genital mutilation and its scope when I read the book *Half the Sky*, by Nicholas Kristof and Sheryl WuDunn.

Years later, in 2012, I began working for Half the Sky Movement, a multimedia project around the book. Here, I was researching organisations and stories on women's oppression around the world, and in part on FGM specifically, for the documentary *Half the Sky*. I was also researching organisations that worked on FGM as on-the-ground partners and activists to be interviewed on film. I have never personally observed or experienced FGM, but it concerns me a great deal.

As part of my Half the Sky Movement work, I was researching and finding anti-FGM non-profit organisations, which we then invited to become our partners. We leveraged footage from the documentary film and via our social media presence to raise awareness about the work of these non-profits and help them reach certain fundraising goals. The storytelling in the film was a powerful way to reach beyond the choir in the USA and internationally to those who knew very little about FGM previously.

The site also hosts blog posts from survivors of and activists around FGM and related issues.

I don't know which are the best ways to eradicate FGM, but one particularly interesting story I have read about came from Tina Rosenberg in *The New York Times*. She details a program in Kembata-Tembaro, Southern Ethiopia, run by FGM survivors Bogaletch Gebre and her sister, which has significantly reduced the support of and incidence of FGM through 'community conversations' or, in more formal parlance, 'deliberative debate'. Its strapline is 'women in Kembata working together'.

Mainstream society must be active in stopping FGM. The practice fundamentally threatens human rights and it deserves the attention of the wider international community. That said however, the international community ought to listen carefully to the voices of those who are affected, at-risk of, or exposed to these practices, because the people who are closest to the issue are those who can best lead the way out.

We must also acknowledge that FGM is not only an issue overseas, but in the 'Western world' as well. It deserves attention at home, in the US and the UK and abroad.

I've been working in journalism for the past four years, in documentary, online and print media. I find that personal storytelling is a powerful way to make change in the campaign against FGM.

I am particularly interested in looking at London neighbourhoods or other English communities where women affected by or are at risk of FGM are campaigning to stop the practice, documenting how they became interested in campaigning against FGM, the work they have been doing, the obstacles they've run into, and the success they have seen.

The media in the UK has done little to capture the human stories of resistance and the tensions between activists campaigning for an end to the practice and supporters of FGM. Exposing how these tensions can develop in communities, and how activists can work to overcome them, is an important solutions angle to contribute to the larger narrative of FGM in the UK.

***

Ms D

I studied, live and now work in London, but in the 1990s, as a teenager, I lived in West Africa (The Gambia). It was then that I first became aware of female genital mutilation.

Some years later, my professional role now includes child protection and work with vulnerable teenagers from the UK and asylum seekers. I have Level 4 child safeguarding training and I am involved weekly with the Child In Need and Child Protection Plans Teams and am part of several core group meetings.

I am currently writing a novel with the purpose of engaging readers of high school and older in understanding exactly what FGM is, how it affects survivors and why it is done. I hope the novel will be a tool to prompt discussion amongst young people in schools and to help professionals identify those at risk.

FGM should become part of the curriculum in high schools and approached in the same manner that sexual exploitation or relationship abuse is discussed. Young women who are survivors going into schools seem to be making quite an impact. This needs to be endorsed and it to be repeated across the country.

Decision makers and the wider community need to be confident that speaking up against FGM isn't being racial or discriminatory against particular communities. It is a human rights issue and all have an equal right to be protected.

It is a non-white practice, but what if the tables were turned? Decision makers need to see the issue aside from the racial boundaries.

We have to recognise and be educated to understand this child abuse issue in line with our own legislation (*Children's Act 1989*). The same applies also for other Western countries such as the USA.

It is difficult for people in traditionally practising communities to speak out, whether in heritage locations or in the diaspora. The spiritual aspects and curses brought upon those who talk about it remain relevant to community members' concerns.

Some progress has been made. The prevalence of FGM in the Mandinka tribe, which I write about, has reduced slightly in the past twenty years. In the mid-1990s it was around 98–99 per cent and now that figure is in the low 90s.

But difficult issues remain. I've recently been involved on Twitter in discussions about the equivalence (or not) of male circumcision (MGM) and FGM. I'm still trying to assess all the information, but I am more inclined than before to see it as a human rights issue. From a Jewish/Christian perspective, I understand from research that the initial type of circumcision was less severe than that practiced nowadays, though I don't know if this is the case.

I wonder if we understand what circumcision actually is? The New Testament says it is a state of people's hearts towards God, a spiritual not physical circumcision. However, unlike FGM, it is a religious requirement for both Muslims and Jews, as well as cultural, which adds a different dynamic. FGM is argued as a religious obligation by many. It isn't, however, referred to in religious texts as specifically as male cutting.

I think there is still scope to change cultural cutting (as opposed to addressing religious circumcision as such) and it is a health issue. Men and boys have also died from the procedure because of infection.

MGM is a topic that needs discussing in line with FGM, especially in communities where it is practised as male circumcision and female 'cutting' is seen as the same thing. If it is OK for the boys, then why not the girls? – I have had such conversations when I lived in Africa.

***

Amanda Epe

I am a British born author and End FGM campaigner of Nigerian heritage. I learnt about FGM as a young adult, when I was told about the practice by my father, who campaigned against it as a teacher in Port Harcourt, Nigeria. I also learnt from my father how it is practised in my Nigerian ethnic community, affecting friends and community members.

Unfortunately FGM is still a secret, and so it is difficult to verify if the practice is diminishing. In the Caribbean I have heard of a practice to keep girls chaste, which seems like a form of female genital destruction where they apply pepper on the female genitals. Women are judged on their sexual health history and rarely freely discuss things openly like men; and sensitive subjects like FGM are really taboo topics in practising communities.

Ever since I heard about FGM, I have been affected. To know of the trauma girls and women have and still face is disturbing, especially when there is denial of the damage, dismissed because it is regarded as a rite of passage.

I liaise in my campaigning against female genital mutilation with Dr Comfort Momoh, a London-based public health specialist for FGM, and other individual activists. I have a blog and project: *Ms Rose Blossom* which is a medium to promote health and literature for girls and women, with a focus on promoting good sexual health and spreading awareness on the physical consequences of FGM, in order to end FGM.

I speak about FGM at community events, to bring about awareness of FGM. This goes beyond targeting groups at risk, because in community events there may be individuals who know someone at risk and but have no prior knowledge of FGM. It has, however, been challenging to do outreach on the ground in formal institutions.

Without a central agency to monitor if schools have had guest speakers giving talks to the pupils I am reluctant to chase up the schools, appearing as a burden, in case they have already involved FGM activists. The schools which need information on FGM the most may also be those least willing to provide it unless they are formally required to do so.

I need support in my work. Individuals such as myself, not set up as charities, must have resources and financial assistance to be empowered in gaining access to schools. There is too much of a top down approach in talking about FGM in the UK. Education authorities should work in collaboration with individuals and organisations.

How the issues are approached is also critical. On occasion I have been contacted by insensitive journalists. A media frenzy sometimes occurs in which they ask me to disclose any traumatic cases of FGM. Language that offends practising communities and sensationalism does not drive the campaign forward.

Further, I believe strongly in more international partnerships.

Nigeria, where my family comes from, has a high incidence of FGM. As the nation has implemented policies to empower women, a national policy to end FGM provides a truly transformational agenda.

To quote the words of Comfort Momoh, 'We need everybody on board the campaign.'

***

Alex Buzzard

It was probably on Twitter about four or five years ago that I first learnt of female genital mutilation, and I have subsequently published a novel, *Consciencia*, on that theme. In my professional name, Ralph Tilby, I have raised matters concerning FGM with the police and other law-makers.

I have a background in management consultancy and have worked with the Metropolitan Police Service. This increased my awareness of just how little priority was given to preventing the abuse of children and in particular preventing FGM. We must make sure the police take the protection of women and children from abuse very seriously.

Having decided I must do something about FGM, I raised an e-petition asking for the Assistant Commissioner of the Metropolitan Police to live up to his responsibilities to protect girls at risk of FGM. The petition raised 1,500 signatures but sadly has had little impact on police performance.

Then in 2014 I lobbied the Home Office Select Committee to investigate why nobody has ever been convicted of FGM and supplied evidence that was mentioned in their report (Ralph Tilby, FGM 0021).

I have also now written a novel, *Consciencia*, which tackles the subject of FGM head on. I have had feedback from a number of different readers who have said the book has made them realise not only the physical impact but the psychological impact of FGM on its victims.

I firmly believe that much of society is protected from the horrors of FGM by the sensitivity of the media. I think there should be some really hard hitting visual images of this practice and more interviews with the victims so that people will engage emotionally with the subject.

Significant impact on progress towards eradicating FGM will demand real change. Police culture is still largely about acquisitive crime, rather than protecting the vulnerable from harm.

....

With Chapter 9 we have reached the end of our global journey behind the curtains of the horrifying worldwide practice of female genital mutilation. This chapter, about the ways that FGM is perceived and the actions taken in the UK, has led us down many different paths. Some of our narrators have chosen to concentrate only on FGM, others have developed interesting and constructive ways to make FGM a focus in the context of their wider professional responsibilities.

Both these approaches provide rich seams to mine, and more about our contributors' endeavours can be learned via the Female Mutilation Worldwide website. One thing is however already clear: all these activities put together offer some very positive routes forward in confronting FGM in the UK, and probably also further afield.

No-one however as yet has the complete answer to how FGM will be eradicated. Our next and final chapter will consider briefly what can be learned from the many and various contributors to this book have so generously shared.

Chapter 10:

What Next?

Our global journey is now done. In our quest to understand female genital mutilation, we have crossed five continents, first of all to Kenya, and then via, other parts of the vast continent of Africa, travelling on to the Middle East and Southeast Asia, and so to Australia. From there we traversed two great oceans, firstly the Pacific to North America, and then the Atlantic to Europe, before arriving finally in the UK, on almost the same time-line as Kenya, where we began.

Had there been the opportunity, we might also have visited secluded communities in South America, for there also female genital mutilation is to be found. FGM recognises few boundaries, whether of geography, nation or tradition.

In one important respect every one of the narratives contained within this book has stood alone. Each person has her or his personal 'story' to tell, and particular ideas to share. The mix is both illuminating and compelling.

It would however be disingenuous to claim that all contributors speak with one voice. On the most important issue of all of course there is unanimity: female genital mutilation is an act of crass cruelty, an abuse which must be stopped. As Dr Morissanda Kouyaté reminds us in his excellent Preface, that is all, when it comes to the fundamentals, which need be said.

Beyond that fundamental unanimity however it is instructive to see on what everyone agrees, and where experience and perspectives diverge.

Yes, everyone concurs, independently across vast divides of context, culture and tradition, that 'education, education, education' must be central to any sort of progress; as must be sincere attempts to work with, not against, the grain of each particular practising community – albeit with a guarantee of direct and serious legal sanction if any child is harmed.

The reports of our correspondents make it clear, however, that unanimity about this general direction of travel must not also be thought to indicate unanimous understandings by the many communities in which it persists about female genital mutilation itself. Whilst each narrative here relates its own realities and understandings, the issues revealed might in general terms be said to cover the basic question of what FGM 'means' to those who perpetuate it, what happens to those who undergo it (and to their communities), who wants to stop it, and what the obstacles and opportunities to achieving that objective might be.

Every reader will have their own appreciations and analysis of what our narrators have so generously revealed; but, as a starting point for those who might find it of interest, we shall identify here briefly some of the general issues.

WHAT DOES FGM 'MEAN'?

Female genital mutilation is chameleon. Its manifest rationales change between locations and over time. For some who promote it, FGM is an act of piety, a way to preserve 'purity' and to hold at bay the otherwise certainty of rampant female teenage sexuality – never mind that testosterone, which might encourage adolescent risk taking, is a male not a female hormone. Science does not play any part in these beliefs. FGM is also for some a trial of things to come. It is a woman's lot – and sometimes via other traditional procedures also a man's – to bear pain, so here's a way to get accustomed to that.

Most overtly, however, as we see when it is re-adopted by isolated groups in the diaspora, FGM denotes membership of the clan or community; and in some instances it denotes too the transition from childhood to 'adulthood' – though sadly not necessarily, given the age of the child at the transition, in any meaningful sense to 'maturity'.

FGM also demonstrates the base, subordinate status of the women in many practising communities. Women are commodities, vessels to produce human resources (babies), to be traded as investments for bride price (dowry) and, for the longer-term, a way of securing their parents' old age via a 'good' (relatively wealthy) 'marriage' (sometimes initially child rape).

But above all FGM signifies power – the absolute authority, even in matters of the utmost personal intimacy, of some people over others. Mostly these powerful people are men, but often it is women who are the functionaries; especially those women who, sanctioned by age-old tradition, secure both income and status from imposing the mutilation that, in an unbreachable conspiracy of silence between them, it is supposed the men of their community require.

This power is patriarchal; that much is evident from the frequently repeated claim that FGM will only stop when the men say it must. The practice is embedded by male decree, in the most literal of ways, into the physical being of girls and young women. By tradition it tolerates no challenge, via either rationality ('FGM isn't good for your health') or any sense of individual autonomy ('I can choose who does what to my body').

There are enormous socio-economic and other practical considerations. How else, as just two examples, will 'professional' mutilators earn their coveted incomes and prestige? What will replace bride price and ancient pension arrangements?

The fundamental position, however, is this:

FGM comprises the ultimate, physical signifier of patriarchy, and of the supremacy of the community over any person in it. Even those who wield this unchallengeable power are however, as some male contributors to this book have told us, constrained by it. No-one may change things, no-one can move beyond the beliefs (and belief traps) that underpin the centrality of genital mutilation.

No wonder FGM is so difficult to erase.

WHAT HAPPENS TO THOSE WHO UNDERGO FGM AND TO THEIR COMMUNITIES?

The stark realities of FGM often remain a mystery to all but initiates, and sometimes even to many who have undergone it. The absolute divisions on many matters between men and women, and the fundamental lack of collective understanding about how anatomy and physiology together determine good health (or not), leave many, often even those who live with FGM, unaware of the damage which it can inflict over a woman's lifetime.

A young girl, 'initiated' and perhaps 'married' to an older man with other wives, may then become a mother (if she lives after giving birth far too early), but she does not thereby become in any meaningful sense mature. Rather, her ostensible gain ('adult' status – even if she is pre-teen) denotes a loss of opportunities, education and autonomy – at least other than exposure to a dangerous level of risky 'choices' within the community itself, now that she is no longer a 'child'. There can be stark outcomes, as we saw in the stories here of sisters who did or did not follow their traditionally determined life course.

Those who are spared or escape the physical harm of FGM are also at risk; their reputations may be in ruins, family relationships destroyed, the security of the group denied to them. Women who do undergo FGM, especially if they were at an age to know about it, often experience not 'only' damage to their bodies, but also damage to their sense of trust and to their peace of mind. How can their mother have permitted this or, at the very least, not prevented it? These are burdensome questions for any child to have to ask.

The damage of FGM to communities is also huge. Healthy girls become to whatever degree incapacitated women, mothers die or are permanently disabled in childbirth, infants (female and male) also die or suffer sometimes permanent injury, resources which could be put to good use are diverted to the direct costs of inflicting mutilation ('celebrations', mutilators' fees etc), educational opportunities diminish and expensive efforts must be invested in combating the practice. These and other adverse impacts, some of them recounted graphically in the narratives in this volume, all hold back communities and economies from delivering a healthier, more positive life for those within them.

WHO WANTS TO STOP FGM? WHAT WILL HINDER OR HELP ERADICATING FGM?

Not only does female genital mutilation take many forms, in many different contexts, but those who oppose it perceive it in different lights as well.

Almost everyone sees FGM firstly as a form of physical harm without benefit (beyond the custom-laden social acceptance it may bring), whoever the perpetrator and whatever the extent or mode of delivery of the damage.

The avoidance of physical risk or harm – to the person concerned and to her future children – stands alone as a reason to challenge FGM, but other considerations often also apply. Amongst these are the psychological and sometimes the socio-economics costs of the mutilation. FGM, as we have seen, fractures trust and relationships, and wastes precious resources. Communities absolutely do not 'need' it. There are other, harmless, ways, as some narrators here have demonstrated, to demark transitions or observe piety, if such must be done.

For some, then, the immediate challenge is the only one: FGM must be stopped because it hurts the people who undergo it, and – where this is also perceived or articulated – the communities it affects. These justifications for eradication stand alone as the basis for opposition to the practice and are, of course, absolutely sufficient in their own right. They are core to the conviction that FGM must stop.

At another level, the perception or choice of rationales for FGM eradication also varies by context and interest or expertise. Whilst individuals directly concerned may articulate their opposition mostly in terms of concerns about damage to the person and to their personal prospects, others may frequently widen the field to include additional forms of harm to (mostly but not always female) children (early marriage, breast ironing, beading, sometimes witchcraft) or to articulate overtly general issues such as violence against women and girls (VAWG), or the principle of human rights.

All these concerns are found to varying degrees in most contexts where FGM occurs, but the emphasis given by different players to each element of the overall rational for opposition often varies; and this is where, as we all seek an end to FGM, the question of 'who does what?' becomes important.

For some grassroots campaigners, it takes all their time and commitment just to insist that FGM is harmful, that it damages people and it must stop. Activists can draw on their close knowledge of immediate context to press compelling arguments against FGM and to urge the adoption of other ways of doing things, replacing the harmful act with other, beneficial ones, perhaps Alternative Rites of Passage (where these apply), and supporting schools and building refuges for girls and young women in peril. Such interventions, often made by individuals, sometimes initially in the face of active opposition or with scant external encouragement, are immensely valuable in their own right.

Other parties, however, must take more formal positions. With just a very small number of exceptions, nations (and religions) around the world have laws against FGM, or at least against hurting people. How these statutes are interpreted is crucial to the likelihood of eradicating FGM in any specific context. That is why getting faith leaders onside is critical in some locations, whilst in others more will be achieved by anyway necessary formal educational, health or legal interventions.

We know that FGM practising communities do not all do it for the same 'reasons' and are not all at the same state of readiness to abandon mutilation. At the local level such considerations are likely to be intrinsically part of activists' strategies, but intervention at more formal levels must be leveraged and calibrated more consciously in these respects. In many cases that will require research and close enquiry at local level. Little will be accomplished in the absence of collaboration with (and active support for) grassroots campaigners on the ground.

Local insights and the efforts of survivors and other resident activists need to be properly respected and sustained by formal agencies working to eradicate FGM. Often however this doesn't happen at any meaningful level, adding yet another cause for concern for campaigners in their own communities who are already seriously burdened.

The situation is more complex when it comes to developing general ways to move forward. Local intelligence, invaluable though it is in that particular locale, may not be very helpful as a more general guide. Laws or, for instance, religious rulings for one sort of community may not be so useful in another. Public health or educational initiatives developed to address a given set of practices may be largely irrelevant elsewhere.

Nor is it always apparent what provision must be made for those who have already undergone FGM. Treatment of the physical harm inflicted must become a priority if those affected are to engage in good health as they would wish in their communities. Restorative surgery is sometimes required but this attention would not initially be welcomed by all. Psychological or social support (remember: all women and girls who have undergone FGM are victims of a serious crime, entitled to reparation for that crime, as well as being 'survivors') may need to be delivered differently in different places, drawing on varied understandings of what has happened.

All this comes before newer issues arising from the debates of modern Western communities can be considered. Can cosmetic surgery, and especially female genital cosmetic surgery, be seen in the same way as FGM? Are those who oppose FGM in the Western world, where there is such an emphasis on manufactured 'beauty', actually hypocrites, and perhaps racist to boot? What about people in many places who are concerned about FGM but ignore male genital mutilation ('MGM', or 'circumcision')? As our commentators have been keen to tell us, child abuse and FGM are everyone's business, but the territory around FGM is not easy to navigate.

BEYOND THE HORROR, TO HOPE

Nonetheless, progress, albeit often far too slowly, is being made.

Cruel and dreadful deeds are still perpetrated and, if we are to make things better, we need to know about them. Little by little, however, the wider context in which these acts occur is changing.

Intermediate technologies have improved beyond anything imaginable even a decade ago. The ways in which people all over the world communicate are now vastly more effective and efficient that before. As one example, many of the contributors to this book were first located via the Internet or simply at random via social media.

The impacts already, and the potential for the future, of the worldwide web and mobile phones are endless. These routes to eradicating FGM and other gendered violence and child abuse or similar hazards are still in their infancy.

The positive potential of the public health approach in such contexts is what must be proclaimed at every possible opportunity. FGM is not 'only' a massive ethics and human rights issues, it is also an enormous challenge to which public health practitioners can and should step up.

FGM is an epidemic of vast proportion. We must never forget that somewhere in the world one more girl is harmed, for her entire life (if she survives the immediate assault), every ten or eleven seconds. Three million women and girls are subjected to FGM every single year. The costs to us all, in resources, in shame, in sheer inhumanity, are beyond comprehension. Good practice in public health can help to make things better.

The same can be said also about education, whether it is targeted at people who need to understand the harms inflicted by specific traditional practices or, much more broadly, at creating a new and brighter world for girls and women, or indeed for entire communities. The eradication of FGM and other traditional human abuses demands a wide-sweeping and positive, multi-faceted approach.

Morissanda Kouyaté, a physician who for decades has been in the vanguard of fighting to stop the massive damage which FGM inflicts, reminds us in his Preface here that it is not simply those immediately involved who must be persuaded to sit up and demand an end to it.

As Executive Director of the Inter-African Committee, Dr Kouyaté drives the eradication of FGM via advocacy and sensitisation, legislation, retraining of excisers, care for victims and networking.

There is no-one reading this book who cannot contribute in some way to at least one of those threads. Every one of us can spread the word and somehow engage with the cause. FGM can and must be stopped, now.

Let's each of us make sure we play our part, whatever that may be, in consigning female genital mutilation to history. Every second and every act of support, however small, really, really matters.

....

For contact details of contributors to this book, and for references and further discussion, please visit the **Female Mutilation Worldwide** *website, at http://femalemutilationworldwide. com/*

INDEX OF CONTRIBUTORS